The
UNBREAKABLE
BRAIN

Shield Your Brain From Cognitive Decline...For Life!

Will Mitchell, LAc, DOM (NM), MS Nutrition

©2015 Primal Health L.P.

DISCLAIMER

This book is intended as reference material, not as a medical manual to replace the advice of your physician or as a substitute for any treatment prescribed by your physician.

If you are ill or suspect that you have a medical problem, we strongly encourage you to consult your medical, health, or other competent professional before adopting any of the suggestions in this book or from drawing inferences from it. If you are taking prescription medication, you should never change your diet or ingest any new supplements without consulting your physician, as any dietary change may alter the effectiveness of that prescription drug and a dietary change may not be appropriate for you.

This book and the author's opinion are for informational and educational purposes only.

The author and publisher of this book and the accompanying materials have used their best efforts in preparing this book. The author and publisher make no representation or warranties with respect to the accuracy, applicability, fitness, or completeness of the contents of this book. The information contained herein is strictly for educational purposes. Therefore, if you wish to apply ideas contained in this book, you are taking full responsibility for your actions. The author and publisher shall in no event be held liable to any party for any direct, indirect, punitive, special, incidental or other consequential damages arising directly or indirectly from any use of this material, which is provided "as is", and without warranties.

CONTENTS

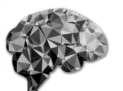

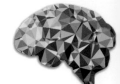

Introduction by Dr. Will Mitchell

One in three people will die of dementia in the United States. Two-thirds of those people are women.

These are terrifying statistics.

Today it's considered normal for people's minds to get weaker, less sharp, and less able as we age. From forgetting where you put your keys to forgetting your children's names, these have become common experiences of aging. Even worse is the growing prevalence of Alzheimer's and other diseases of dementia. They cause millions of people to suffer as they lose their autonomy, freedom, and independence bit by bit.

You may be wondering what you can do to avoid becoming one of those individuals. Is it possible to prevent dementia? Or reverse it?

The answer is yes. While the brain may still hold some mysteries, there is a lot we do know about getting and keeping it healthy and reversing the damage that might already be there. Your brain is the interface between your mind and spirit in this world, but it is also a physical organ that, like all organs, has nutritional needs and chemical stresses. Just like keeping a body physically fit requires exercise and nutritious food, a brain needs to be fed and exercised to stay strong or get stronger.

I invite you to consider that we have discovered tools and mechanisms that can keep a brain healthy and sharp. If you think this is impossible, or a pipe dream, read on:

In a fall 2014 press release, Dr. Dale Bredesen said:

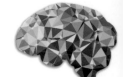

The existing Alzheimer's drugs affect a single target, but Alzheimer's disease is more complex. Imagine having a roof with 36 holes in it, and your drug patched one hole very well. The drug may have worked, and a single hole may have been fixed, but you still have 35 other leaks, and so the underlying process may not be affected much.[1]

His point was that Alzheimer's is a disease in which multiple factors — inflammation, poor blood sugar, poor nutrition, life stresses, etc. — all come together to form a single terrible result. So unlike with existing therapies, which just address one of those factors, he wanted to see what would happen if he patched as many of those holes as he could.

Bredesen designed a study that did exactly that, putting ten people with varying degrees of cognitive decline on a multi-faceted regime:[2] It started with managing their blood sugar, eating a low glycemic, low grain, low inflammatory diet. They took out processed foods and added in fresh vegetables, fruits, and healthy meats (as naturally raised or organic as possible). He had them incorporate stress reduction in the form of yoga or meditation. He made sure they got eight hours of sleep per night, and that they exercised 30–60 minutes per day, 4–6 times per week. They took B vitamins, and herbs like ginkgo, ashwaganda and bacopa, and made sure their vitamin D levels were optimal. They took supplements like zinc and copper, CoQ10, and carnitine. If they had sleep apnea, they were treated for it. They ate medium chain triglyceride oil. And more. All in all, they (and their caretakers) did a lot of stuff.

Here's what happened (and this may blow your mind):

One 67-year old patient had been doing terribly at work. She would get lost driving, and forget where her exits were. She forgot what she had read by the time she got to the bottom of a page. She mixed up the names of her pets, and couldn't remember where the light switches were in the house that she had lived in for years. Her mother had died of dementia, and her doctor had told her she had the same condition.

Though she was only able to take on some of the suggestions, within three months:

> "She was able to navigate without problems, remember telephone numbers without difficulty, prepare reports and do all of her work without difficulty, read and retain information, and, overall, she became asymptomatic. She noted that her memory was now better than it had been in many years. On one occasion, she developed an acute viral illness, discontinued the program, and noticed a decline, which reversed when she reinstated the program. Two and one-half years later, now age 70, she remains asymptomatic and continues to work full-time."

Also in the study was a 55-year old attorney who had suffered with severe memory issues — she had left the stove on multiple times, forgot meetings and scheduled multiple meetings at the same time, took copious notes on her iPad so as to not forget things but then forgot the password to her iPad. She was unable to do her job and was considering leaving.

After five months on the program, she no longer needed her iPad to take notes and no longer forgot conversations. She went back to work, started to learn Spanish, and began a new legal specialty. Her children noted that she no longer became lost mid-sentence, no longer thought she had asked them to do something that she had not asked, and answered their questions with normal speed and memory.

Overall, Dr. Bredesen's study had a 90% improvement rate, meaning that nine of the ten participants saw distinct, sustainable, and noticeable changes in their cognition. Only one of them — who had advanced Alzheimer's disease — did not improve.

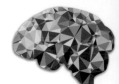

That's nine people who would have stopped recognizing their family and friends; who would have had to stop doing what they loved; who would have gone on to spend years declining in a nursing home, all reversed because they took on their health in a massive way.

If they could do it, and cause such huge improvement, you can too. You just have to start, and we're here to help.

If you are reading this then I know that you are up for the task.

Chapter 1: Brain 101

Understanding how the brain works

The brain is a unique and fascinating organ. It performs more distinct and simultaneous functions than anything else in the body, keeping our lungs breathing, our hearts beating, our intestines moving, our body temperatures regulated, our immune systems functioning, and more — and it does all of those things without us even paying attention. Then there are the parts we actually notice happening — consciously moving our bodies and thinking — which are equally miraculous.

Our brains are uniquely organized to manage all these tasks. As babies, they're like a giant pile of wires and transistors. At first there are comparatively few connections between each of those parts, but the number of potential connections is astronomical. Then every time we learn something, our brains connect this wire to that wire, that wire to that transistor, and so on, forming a growing number of complex circuits that we call memories, habits, reflexes, thoughts, emotions, talents, and so on.

The important part of this equation is not the number of parts (called **neurons**, and sometimes referred to as **gray matter**), or the size of the brain, but rather the number of connections (called **synapses** and **dendrites**, often referred to as **white matter**) being made. When you think about what a brain looks like, the reason for all those wrinkles and folds is to maximize the number of potential connections. Albert Einstein had his brain examined after he passed away,

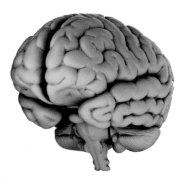

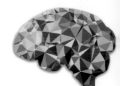

and it turns out that his brain actually weighed less than average but the number of connections was immense!

So since that's the subject of the hour — what causes our brains to stop working properly, and what we can do to fix it — let's look at how it works.

The Working Brain

Obviously, the brain is a very specialized organ, and the one that set us apart from all other animals. We have hinged joints in our skull so that babies' large heads can fit through the birth canal when we're born. The brain uses 87% of an 8 lb baby's metabolism.[3] Even as adults it uses 25% of our metabolism[4] — which is pretty impressive, considering it comprises just 1–2% of our body weight.

I'm not going to go into a lot of detail here about who does what in the brain. Partly that's because it's mind-bogglingly complicated (no pun intended), but second it's because scientists barely know how it all ties together.

But to give you a very crude crash course, there are three main parts to the brain:

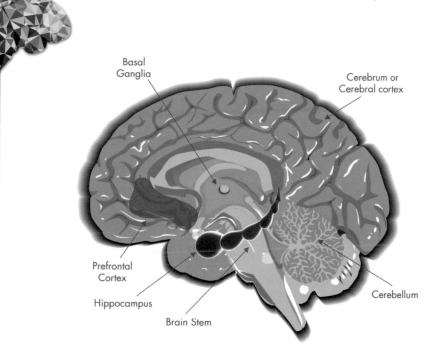

Basal
Ganglia

Cerebrum or
Cerebral cortex

Prefrontal
Cortex

Hippocampus

Brain Stem

Cerebellum

- The **BRAIN STEM** controls our most basic brain function: the autonomic systems. This includes breathing, digestion, heartbeat, etc. — the things that run on their own, whether you want them to or not.

- The **CEREBELLUM** mostly controls our physical movements (i.e., balance and motor control). It serves some cognitive functions too, though — mostly ones that are associated with repetition and automatic responses like language, emotions (fear/pleasure), and so-called procedural memories (things like riding a bike, tying a shoelace, or reading).

- The **CEREBRUM** or **CEREBRAL CORTEX** makes up about three-quarters of a human's brain (much more than any other animal), and although it serves some of those autonomic functions, too, this is where the bulk of cognitive activity takes place, including sensory perception, conscious thought, and memory retention. It has a number of different sub-sections, but perhaps the parts most critically associated with memory are include:

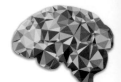

- The **PREFRONTAL CORTEX**, right behind your forehead, which stores short-term and long-term memories; and

- The **LIMBIC SYSTEM**, in the middle of the brain, which plays a number of key roles in processing memories. Particularly noteworthy parts of the limbic system are:

  - The **HIPPOCAMPUS**, which converts short-term into long-term memories; and

  - The **BASAL GANGLIA**, which has a section called the striatum important in forming and retrieving procedural memories.

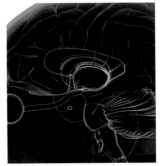

As I said, this all ties together in incredibly complex ways. For example, the limbic system is actually composed of more than a dozen distinct structures that serve a number of primary roles related to emotions and behavior. But most of those structures are also involved in memory function one way or another. Every piece of a memory is stored in the section of the brain specific to that kind of experience, so although, for example, the amygdala controls fight or flight, that emotional response is often the result of historical incidents (you got bitten by a spider, now you're afraid of spiders), which are stored in the amygdala and then retrieved when necessary. If you think about the last meal you ate, the taste memory is stored in the taste section of the brain, what it looked like is stored in the optical section of the brain, how you felt about that meal is stored in the emotions section of the brain, and so on. Then it's the hippocampus that connects all those individual memories together to form a single episode.

All of which is to say, the brain is way too complex to simply point to the part that controls memory and say, "Look, there it is!" It's a dense and highly connected web that processes countless pieces of information at once. And here's why this is important: because of how interconnected it is, the brain needs a highly efficient communication system in order to do its job properly.

That communication system comes in the form of **neurotransmitters** — chemicals that literally transmit information from one part the brain to another. You may have heard names like serotonin or dopamine, our brain's natural "happy chemicals." These are neurotransmitters — they are manufactured and formed in one section of the brain, and then released to travel to another part of the brain to produce a distinct experience or emotion.

It turns out, both serotonin and dopamine affect memory in ways we'll get to later. Other neurotransmitters involved in memory, learning, attention, and wakefulness (which are all connected to the memory system) include:

- ACETYLCHOLINE, which is primarily associated with other functions, but also impacts attention and concentration;

- GLUTAMATE, the most abundant neurotransmitter in the nervous system, and which does the actual work of strengthening the synapses between the pre-frontal cortex and the hippocampus (forming those long-term memories);

- EPINEPHRINE, more commonly known as adrenaline, which strengthens memory connections during stressful situations so that the strength of a memory is proportional to its importance; and

- NOREPINEPHRINE which has been found to stimulate the hippocampus for spatial memory retrieval (in other words, remembering where you are and where you are going).[5]

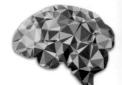

When the System Breaks

Unlike all other tissues in the body, our neurons do not store any energy themselves. The complete running out of energy causes cells to die, which is why every other cell in the body has enough energy stored up that it can survive for hours outside the body if placed on ice. But the brain needs to be fed constantly by the blood vessels around it, and it needs a constant supply of oxygen, or else the neurons will die.

In fact, brains are so sensitive that even minor drops in blood sugar or oxygen can significantly reduce their functionality — leading to symptoms like fatigue, an inability to concentrate, and irritability or other mood changes. (Sound familiar?) More severe drops in blood sugar or oxygen lead to unconsciousness — the body can't survive without the brain, so if there's not enough energy to feed it, it shuts down all the systems it needs to in order to keep the brain running a little while longer.

In addition to all of that, your brain needs access to the proper ingredients in order to perform all its myriad functions. Long term memories are made with the production of new proteins, which requires minerals like calcium and magnesium. Serotonin, dopamine, and glutamate are made from amino acids. Acetylcholine is made from choline, a B vitamin (found in liver and egg yolks). There are more than a hundred neurotransmitters known so far, and the basic message is the same: they are all made from nutrients.

But wait, there's more. Anything that your body is exposed to for a long period of time, it will adapt to accommodate. If you stare at a bright light for fifteen minutes and then look away, you'll have a hard time seeing for a little while, right? Now imagine staring at that bright light for twenty years. How long do you think it'll take before you can see properly? Days? Months? Years? Never?

The same thing happens in our bodies: when they're constantly exposed to certain stressors, they acclimate and/or become damaged over time. For example, cortisol is the hormone our bodies release during stress. The hippocampus has many cortisol receptors, which is why people are often able to remember so much detail about highly stressful situations (e.g., a car crash) — the stress receptors flood into the hippocampus at the same time as the incident, producing a highly detailed memory. However, too much cortisol over time damages the hippocampus in the same way that too much light exposure damages the eyes, which in turn damages our ability to recall long term (and sometimes short term) memories. And humans these days are constantly exposing ourselves to stress.

So the upshot is this: When the brain lacks the ability to retrieve energy from the blood vessels, it can't do its job properly and can get damaged. When it lacks the ability to retrieve oxygen from the blood vessels, it can't do its job properly and can get damaged. When it lacks sufficient nutrients it can't do its job properly. When it's exposed to too much stress it can get damaged.

Alzheimer's, effectively, is the result of one or more of the above occurring over a long period of time. In various parts of the brain (most notably the cerebrum and the hippocampus), plaques build up and neural fibers get "tangled,"[6] breaking the communication system and resulting in the slow and steady death of the neurons and synapses. Those sections then atrophy, leading to memory problems and, eventually, disorientation, speech problems, behavioral issues and all the other symptoms we associate with Alzheimer's and dementia.[7]

And although "pruning" is a normal part of brain function — unneeded neurons die off all the time, so that the body doesn't have to waste energy feeding cells that it doesn't need — obviously we want our brains to be smart about the neurons it chooses to kill off. That's why it's so important how you use and feed those neurons. Which is really what this book is about.

Chapter 2: Risk Factors

Doctors and scientists have spent a lot of time trying to figure out what causes Alzheimer's and dementia, just as they have trying to figure out what causes any number of other diseases. In theory, anywhere in life we can determine that A causes B, all we have to do to stop B from happening is to eliminate A.

Unfortunately, human beings aren't quadratic equations. We can't just solve for x. Everyone is different, and even if we feed two different people the exact same things, or give them the exact same stressors, their bodies will respond differently. So the best we can do is make educated guesses as to what can increase your risk.

In general, the risk for dementia is age related, not gender related.[8] However, women with two genetic copies of the e4 variation of the APOE gene (we'll talk about that below) have double the risk of men,[9]

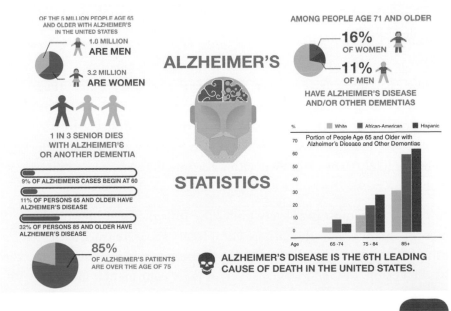

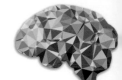

and there is some evidence that this happens more often to women, depending on what you read. Ninety percent of Alzheimer's occurs after 60 years old, but new cases are not common after 90. It is twice as common in African-Americans as in Caucasian-Americans.[10]

However, if we're trying to guess at what causes Alzheimer's, there are a number of things we can point to, particularly in the way of medical issues and lifestyle/environmental factors that can increase your risk. And that's mainly what this chapter is focused on.

Medical Issues

Our culture as a whole is pretty terrible at preventive medicine. What we typically think of as "preventive" is really just early detection. While it's true that early screening through tests like pap smears and digital prostate exams have saved thousands of lives, they're still not preventing any diseases so much as catching them early enough that the treatment will be more effective. *True prevention* requires making lifestyle choices that keep those diseases from showing up in the first place. And we're terrible at that.

The reason is because we don't think of cancer, or diabetes, or heart disease as an immediate concern. It's some theoretical problem that happens to other people, but *I'm* not going to get it. A survey from Aflac insurance[11] found that 62% of American workers said they were not likely to be diagnosed with a serious illness like cancer; 55% said they were not likely to be diagnosed with a chronic illness like heart disease or diabetes.

Added to that, most people are under the mistaken assumption that mental and physical ailments are completely separate from each other. They think that if you develop diabetes, or heart disease, or hypertension, or God forbid, cancer, at least your mental faculties will be the same. You'll still have your wits about you, so you'll be able to approach those conditions thoughtfully and treat them intelligently.

Unfortunately, these people are in for a rude awakening. The reality about chronic diseases is just the opposite of what the American public thinks: they account for 7 of the 10 leading causes of death in the United States comprising some two-thirds of all deaths.[12] And study after study proves that if you *do* end up with any of these diseases, it's not long before cognitive changes set in.

Heart Disease

Let's start with America's number one killer. It should come as no surprise that dementia can be caused by **strokes** (or a series of small strokes), **atherosclerosis** (plaque build-ups in the blood vessels) causing blockages in the brain, and **inflammation** from things like smoking, brain injuries, or hypertension. All of these damage blood vessels in the brain, leading to less-than-optimal brain function.

More than twenty years ago researchers were noting that plaques in the carotid arteries and elsewhere all contributed to cognitive decline in older people,[13] and the research has only expanded since then. A recent study examined the brains of 69 patients at risk of developing dementia, starting in their 30s, then 21 years later, and then again 7 years after that. Patients with heart disease had a thinner brain cortex and less gray matter, and the longer the patients had the heart disease, the worse it got. This was especially true in those who had heart disease for more than 10 years.[14]

Another study looked at men aged 40 to 80, and they saw that, compared to men with no heart disease, those with subclinical or prevalent heart disease all had lower scores on memory performance and lower scores on processing capacity and executive functioning.[15] In fact, their conclusion

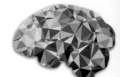

stated, "These results suggest that actions to prevent cognitive decline by preventing atherosclerosis should be taken before middle age" — yet another voice for prevention, rather than just early detection.

What about other heart issues? Growing evidence now links **atrial fibrillation** (irregular heart beat) with significant cognitive decline through a number of different pathways: a German study that demonstrated people with AF performed significantly worse in tasks of learning, memory, attention, and executive functions, with a corresponding degeneration of the hippocampus (a part of the brain that plays a crucial role in memory function).[16]

And of course, atrial fibrillation may lead to heart attacks, strokes, and embolisms (blood clots) — which, as you now know, can cause further cognitive problems. Atrial fibrillation will be diagnosed in 25% of people over 40 years old.

Hypertension, or high blood pressure, literally means that the pressure the blood is exerting on the vessels is higher than it should be. And just like excessive tire pressure can damage a car's tires, and high water pressure can damage the pipes in your home, high blood pressure damages the blood vessels.

In the brain specifically, hypertension damages the cerebral arteries, which leads to brain atrophy and lesions.[17] It's long been known that high blood pressure leads to cognitive impairment, and the reverse is also true: when people with hypertension are able to manage their blood pressure and keep it managed, their chances of brain problems go down.[18]

All of which is to say, if you have any kind of health problems that fall under the broad umbrella of heart disease, you're at much greater risk of cognitive decline, too.

Diabetes

Did you ever think that having diabetes would make you more prone to develop dementia?

The connection between the two is now so strong that Alzheimer's disease is starting to be referred to as "Type 3 Diabetes."[19,20] And you don't have to get diagnosed with diabetes for this to be an issue — long before that, the years of high blood sugar have an impact on brain function.

High blood sugar causes insulin resistance of the brain, which has been implicated in the formation of the amyloid plaques associated with Alzheimer's. Having diabetes can more than *double* your chances of getting Alzheimer's, and there's evidence that the chances of developing some form of dementia (including but not limited to Alzheimer's) can be as high as 74% for diabetics.[21]

The biggest influences on why brain functions decline in diabetics has to do with poor blood sugar control, high blood sugar, inflammation, depression, and problems with the capillaries (the smallest blood vessels), which can get so damaged as to start to disintegrate as the disease progresses.

Additionally, diabetics often have high blood pressure, heart disease, and kidney problems, which bring their own risks to cognitive health.

Scientists see a clear correlation between dementia and Type 2 diabetes and are now calling it an epidemic. They report that diabetes is a known risk factor for the development of dementia due to clogged arteries, Alzheimer's disease, and cognitive impairment. The types of cognitive impairment seen in diabetics include decreases in attention span, executive functions, psychomotor speed, and memory. We mentioned "executive functions" before — it refers to a category of brain functions that involve working memory, flexibility, reasoning, planning, problem solving and execution. Psychomotor speed is the amount of time from when you get an idea to move your muscles to the time that the action of your muscles is initiated. For example, you see a cup of coffee and want to pick it up to drink it. Psychomotor speed is the time it takes you to go from idea to action.

Japanese scientists found that 72% of the Type 2 diabetics in their study also had a dysfunction in their frontal lobe (the part of the brain responsible for muscle movement, attention, planning, motivation, and short-term memory) and recall memory. They believe that diabetes may be linked not only to Alzheimer's disease but also to Parkinson's disease, Huntington's disease and frontotemporal lobe dementia.[22]

Depression

People sometimes manifest dementia-like symptoms — forgetfulness, disorientation, inattentiveness, and slowed responses — when they are depressed. Conversely, having some cognitive decline can *cause* depression.

Researchers don't necessarily know yet what the mechanism of action is, but they have seen some interesting facts. For example, in people with mild cognitive impairment (a transitional state between normal aging and dementia) those who also had depression were more than twice as likely to develop dementia of Alzheimer's type. Those who did not respond well to antidepressants were at an especially increased risk of developing dementia.[23]

While researchers are working to unravel the association between depression and cognitive decline, the best thing to do in the meantime is to take active steps to handle any depression that might be there.

Pernicious Anemia/Vitamin B12 Deficiency

Vitamin B12 is vital for the nervous system to act properly, so it's possible to get dementia-like symptoms if you have pernicious anemia, or B12 deficiency. This is very common in the elderly due to lack of absorption, not eating enough meat or eggs, or as a side effect of certain medications.

Symptoms of B12 deficiency include confusion, slowness, irritability, and apathy, as well as loss of balance, and numbness and tingling. Fortunately, this is a condition that can easily be detected through a simple blood test, and it's a simple treatment through B12 supplementation.

Lifestyle and Environmental Factors

The reality of the medical issues described above is that, generally speaking, they are the result of a long series of lifestyle choices that were going on for decades before any symptoms started to show up. We live in a culture where processed foods are cheap, 60+-hour work weeks are plentiful, a full night's sleep is scarce, and exercise is inconvenient. Our bodies were never built to withstand that kind of stress, and after years of dealing with it, these are the results.

Not surprisingly, the same factors that lead to those medical issues like heart disease and diabetes can directly lead to Alzheimer's, even in the absence of other medical problems.

Diet

You may remember that Bredesen, in the study I talked about in the Introduction, had his patients make some rather significant changes to their diets — taking away processed foods, adding in vegetables, fruits, and naturally raised meats, eating organic as much as possible, and emphasizing low glycemic, low grain, low inflammatory foods. There was a reason for all of these things.

Much of the research on diet, nutrition, and disease that has come out in the last couple of decades has pointed to a simple truth: that one way or another, inflammation is the source of most of our modern diseases.

- Poor blood sugar, as we talked about in the Diabetes section above, leads to insulin resistance, which causes inflammation.
- Fake food that is manufactured in a lab by chemical engineers, rather than grown directly out of the ground, causes inflammation.
- Antibiotics, which are injected indiscriminately into our livestock, cause inflammation.
- Toxins, which are plentiful in our food thanks to the unrelenting use of pesticides, cause inflammation.

With any or all of these, plaques can build up in the brain, which impairs the neurons' ability to communicate with each other. Then, because we're not eating well, our bodies lack the proper nutrients to break these plaques down, which further perpetuates the problem and turns it into a vicious circle.

When all of this happens, impaired cognition is an obvious result.

All of which is to say that your risk of Alzheimer's is significantly higher if you eat:

- Processed foods,
- Conventionally grown (non-organic) red meat and vegetables,
- Lots of sugar,
- Lots of grains, starches, and other high-glycemic foods.

Stress

Stress does indeed damage the brain.[24] Most noticeably it causes high cortisol which, over time, atrophies the hippocampus and our memories. This has been observed in brain studies of adults with Post Traumatic Stress Disorder (PTSD) and in children who were abused. It has also been replicated in controlled studies with primates. In rats the same damage has been studied from exposure to prolonged stress and they found free radical damage to fats in the cerebral cortex, cerebellum, hippocampus, and midbrain. Protein damage from oxidation were also found in the cortex, hypothalamus, striatum, and medulla oblongata.[25]

Stress not only ages our brains, but even shortens our telomeres. Telomeres[26] are the sequences at the end of our chromosomes that protect the chromosome from aging — a bumper, if you will, that's designed to get worn down. Essentially, they regulate our lifespan, and as we age, they shorten. So stress literally ages us and damages our DNA if we don't manage it.

Sleep

Sometimes people question the wisdom in "sleeping a third of your life away," but now we know that sleep is the only way to restore your brain function to 100%. Sleep is important for memory consolidation (moving memories from short-term into long-term storage), clearing metabolic waste from the brain, body growth/repair in general, behavior/moods, and there's no shortage of studies showing how sleep impacts cognition. There's even evidence now that our bodies activate different genes when we're asleep than when we're awake.[27]

It naturally follows that when we're not sleeping as much as our bodies need, it causes diminished function in the body and brain in any number of ways. These include:

- obvious effects like fatigue, and difficulty concentrating;
- diminished cognitive function,[28] which includes impairments to learning, memory, speed, and verbal tasks; and
- significant reductions in overall health, with symptoms including immune function decline,[29] cancer,[30] reduced mineral density,[31] hypertension,[32] and an inability to process carbohydrates,[33] which can cause weight gain[34] and its corresponding concerns relating to heart disease and blood sugar/diabetes..

And these symptoms only get worse as sleep debt builds.[35]

Because sleep affects your brain, we often can't tell when we're having symptoms of sleep deprivation. In other words, we lose touch with what normal thinking and brain function feels like and we think our current mental state is normal.

Sleep is so important that we wrote a whole bonus report on it, so please read that for more information.

And for the record, depression is something that can absolutely impact sleep. When people are depressed they may have low serotonin — which everyone knows as the neurotransmitter that helps with moods and thinking, but another one of its crucial functions is to make melatonin, the neurotransmitter that helps us sleep. So low serotonin means low melatonin, and the result is difficulty sleeping.

Smoking

Anything that reduces oxygen to your brain is going to increase your risk of cognitive decline, and the fact that smoking does that is a no-brainer. (Haha! See what I did there?) Smoking increases your risk of Alzheimer's by 45%,[36] and 14% of all Alzheimer's cases can be directly attributed to smoking.[37]

And unfortunately, it has an impact far beyond the immediate and obvious. A large, multi-ethnic study published in 2011[38] explored the impact mid-life smoking had on dementia diagnoses decades later, and what they saw was that people who were heavy smokers in the middle of their lives basically doubled their incidence of dementia and Alzheimer's later in life.

And if you have high blood sugar *and* you smoke, your risk for cognitive decline only gets worse,[39] as diabetes damages the blood vessels in the brain. It's no surprise that adding smoking to this picture causes so much injury.

Exercise (or Lack Thereof)

We've already talked about how diabetes, hypertension, heart disease and other medical issues impact dementia. And we've talked about how diet impacts dementia directly, and everyone knows that diet impacts those health concerns.

It follows naturally that the flip side of that equation, exercise, also impacts dementia, and indeed the research bears that out. People who don't exercise are more likely to develop dementia or Alzheimer's. Women are nearly twice as likely to develop it without exercise.[40]

It actually has such an association that a study titled "Lack of exercise is a major cause of chronic diseases"[41] goes into heavy detail about the impact

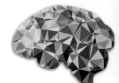

of lack of exercise on every chronic health condition we see these days. It even showed that mice with a genetic propensity toward cognitive decline could reverse it, with exercise, to the levels of mice without that genetic defect.

We'll talk much more about this in later chapters when we talk about the *benefits* to exercise. For now, just be aware that lack of exercise contributes to Alzheimer's every bit as much as it contributes to cardiovascular disease.

Toxins

We are starting to see a clear picture that we are surrounded by toxins, and most everything that is toxic to our bodies will eventually affect our most complex organ.

Pesticides like DDT, which is still in our environment, are much higher in the brains of people with Alzheimer's. Although there are genetic risks to getting the disease, these do not explain the high prevalence of Alzheimer's today and scientists are concerned that modern toxins like DDT are a big factor.[42]

Aluminum is another toxin that has been associated with Alzheimer's for decades now,[43] and the more research is done on the subject the more it appears that the two are linked.[44] Obvious aluminum sources include aluminum pots and pans, antiperspirants, antacids, vaccines, aluminum foil and soda or food cans.

Toxins called nitrosamines, which come from meats cooked at high temperatures, have also been linked to Alzheimer's.[45] The common use of nitrogen-containing compounds (nitrates and nitrites as preservatives) along with cooking methods (e.g., grilling) that bind the nitrogen to amino acids in protein foods is causing more stress on our bodies. This stress to our arterial lining, the endothelium, increases our insulin resistance and thus Alzheimer's. (Actually, anything that damages the capillaries, or microcirculation, can reduce brain volume, specifically white matter.)[46]

Then there's fluoride toxicity. The pineal gland, located just behind your forehead, is where melatonin is made, and this gland is sensitive to fluoride, collecting more than any other part of the body. After too much fluoride the pineal glands calcify — which has an obvious impact on the production of melatonin, and in turn, your ability to sleep. To some extent pineal gland calcification is a normal part of aging, but it's also been linked to Alzheimer's[47] and other diseases. Where do we get fluoride from? Antidepressant drugs like Prozac (⅓ fluoride by weight), fluoride-based antibiotics like Cipro, cooking with Teflon, and of course it's added to our water supply.

Even air pollution has been studied and found to increase Alzheimer's.[48]

Besides taking normal precautions to avoid unnecessary exposure to toxins, good nutrition is how our bodies clean themselves. We'll get to that in later chapters.

Genetics

The APOE gene deals with cholesterol production and transport, and it's called a "risk-factor gene" because a certain variation of it (APOEe4 allele or genetic version) increases a person's risk of developing cardiovascular disease and Alzheimer's. Approximately 14% of the Caucasian population and 19% of people of African descent have the APOEe4 version.

Here's the thing, though — just because the two are associated does *not* mean that APOEe4 *causes* Alzheimer's. People get Alzheimer's who have a different strain of APOE, and there are people with APOEe4 who

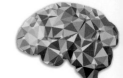

don't get Alzheimer's at all. It simply means that the risk may be greater, especially with certain other factors added.

Scientists are beginning to realize that it's really a combination of multiple genes, lifestyle, and stressors that cause disease. Just like it's not a single gene, but a combination of many genes and lifestyle factors (diet, exercise, etc.) that gives someone NBA basketball height, diseases are caused by a combination of genes, sometimes thousands of them, working in concert with *epigenetic factors* (outside influences like diet, exercise, chemicals, smoking, certain nutrients, or stress) that turn those genes on or off.

This is why people even in the same family will not all have the same health issues. And it's also why genetic testing for Alzheimer's is not recommended.[49] Regardless of what your genes say or don't say, there are steps to take to prevent and reverse cognitive decline.

Easily Reversible Causes of Dementia

Before moving on, it's worth noting that there are four easily reversible causes of dementia:

* **HYPOTHYROIDISM** – A deficiency in the ability of the thyroid to produce important hormones.
* **VITAMIN B12 DEFICIENCY** – We'll talk more about this in chapter 6.
* **LYME DISEASE** – A tick-borne bacterial illness that causes inflammation and neurological problems. People who spend a lot of time in tall grasses and heavily-wooded areas are at higher risk. In addition to memory loss, symptoms may include joint pain, numb or weak limbs, depression, partial facial paralysis, fatigue, and more.

- NEUROSYPHILIS – The result of syphilis left untreated for many years, at which point the disease spreads to the brain and spinal cord.

All people with memory difficulties should get tested for thyroid function and B12 deficiency, as these are easily detectable and easily reversible. The other two should be tested for as well if there are risk factors involved.

Chapter 3: Your Brain On Drugs

Did you know that prescription drugs could actually be a cause of memory loss or other cognitive deficits? There are tons of drugs out there that alter neurotransmitters, which causes problems with brain health sooner later. There are drugs that can deplete B vitamins. And there are others, too.

So it might not be you who is declining mentally; your medications could be at fault.

Before we go any further, it's important to reiterate that you should *never stop taking prescription medications without the express recommendation of your doctor*. If you're on one of these medications and think it could be having a negative effect, talk to your doctor and see what alternatives are available to you.

Antidepressants

There are several different classes of antidepressants. The ones that seem to be the worst for memory function are tricyclic antidepressants, which include Sinequan, Tofranil, Elavil, Pamelor, Vivactil, Anafranil, Triavil, Asendin, Limbitrol and Norpramin. These drugs are anticholinergic, meaning that they interfere with acetylcholine, the most important neurotransmitter for thinking.[50] Just over half of people taking these drugs will experience loss of concentration. About 35% will say they have memory impairment.

For the record, you don't need to have depression to be prescribed tricyclic antidepressants. Eating disorders, chronic pain, menstrual cramps, obsessive-compulsive disorder, and even hormonal issues like hot flashes can spur your doctor to prescribe these medications.

Selective Serotonin Inhibitors (SSRIs) are another common class of antidepressants, and these have been found to impair episodic memory[51] — the memory of details of events in your life. This is the exact memory you would use to write your autobiography. SSRIs also change the dendrite connections between neurons in your brain, especially in the cortex (your conscious thinking), a phenomenon that has been measured within three hours of the first dose.[52] If you recall from the beginning of this book, Einstein was a genius because of the tremendous of connections in his cortex. While the drug companies go on about increased axon growth (one end of the neurons), they leave out this detail about the dendrite connections.

Lithium — which is used for regulating bipolar mood swings — is also associated with cognitive dysfunctions.[53]

Diabetes Medications

Of course, we've already talked about how diabetes can lead to dementia, but some of the medications that reduce blood glucose cause cognitive decline all on their own. Metformin is one example, ostensibly by causing B12 and other vitamin deficiencies.[54]

Cholesterol-Lowering Medications

Statins are notorious for causing severe memory loss.

There are different types of statins on the market, such as Zocor, Crestor, Lipitor, Pravachol, and Lescol. These drugs work by lowering the amount of cholesterol that is produced in the body.

Although your doctor may think this is vital, there are some serious ramifications. For example, cholesterol is used in your body as a precursor compound for different hormones and even for a chemical your body synthesizes called dolichol. This chemical is essential for your memory but it doesn't get created when cholesterol synthesis is blocked. Cholesterol is also important for the connections between nerve cells.

One University of California San Diego study surveyed 171 patients between the ages of 34 and 86 years old to discover how frequently memory and other cognitive problems resulted after taking statins. Seventy-five percent of them experienced negative changes in cognitive functioning. Eighty-four percent of them stopped statin therapy, and 90% of them reported an improvement in their brain functioning within about two and a half weeks. Some patients who had been diagnosed with Alzheimer's or dementia had their diagnosis reversed.[55] When 19 patients started up on statins again, the same cognitive deficits show up.

Since 2009 the FDA has required statins to include a warning about possible memory problems.

Drugs to Reduce Blood Pressure

Beta-blockers are commonly prescribed for congestive heart failure, arrhythmia, high blood pressure and fast heart rate as well as migraines and angina. Lopressor, Toprol, Coreq, Tenormin, Betapace, and Inderal are some of the more common ones. These drugs cause memory problems by preventing the neurotransmitters epinephrine and norepinephrine from retrieving memory, especially in patients who already have some cognitive decline.[56]

Parkinson's Medications

As a disease of the brain, Parkinson's is treated with many medications that alter the production or elimination of neurotransmitters. There are

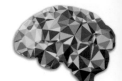

drugs that increase dopamine (L-DOPA, Mirapex, Requip, Parlodel, and Apokyn), which is needed for thinking, pleasure, and initiation of movement. There are anticholinergic medications (Scopolamine, Atropine), which block the neurotransmitter acetylcholine, inhibiting parasympathetic nerve impulses but also directly impairing thinking.

Other Parkinson's medications block COMT or MAO, enzymes that break down neurotransmitters and keep the brain going. These include Tasmar (anti-COMT), Eldepryl (anti-MAO), Stalevo (combo, anti-COMT), Comtan (anti-COMT), and Cogentin (anticholinergic).

In other words, some of the Parkinson's medications handle a symptom while creating more cognitive decline. As a recent editorial to the American Academy of Family Physicians put it, "Clinicians should evaluate patients for other causes of dementia, and consider discontinuing anticholinergic or dopaminergic medications that may contribute to cognitive impairment."[57]

Narcotic Painkillers

The list of narcotics is quite long: Butorpanol, Fentanyl, Demerol, Talwin, Tramadol, Vicodin, Norco, Dilaudid, Exalgo, Oxycontin, Avinza, Percocet, and Astramorph are some of the ones that are commonly prescribed for use at home. However, the list doesn't stop there. There are also combination pain drugs that include a narcotic ingredient — for example, acetaminophen combined with codeine to make hydrocodone or oxycodone; or aspirin and oxycodone mixed together to make Percodan.

Narcotics are derived from opium, which acts on the nervous system by stopping your emotional reaction to pain and interrupting the flow of pain signals, making you sleepy and unresponsive to the pain. The pain is still there, but you become unable to care about it. If that is how you react to pain, just imagine how poor your focus on everyday tasks will be on narcotics. The result is a change in short-term and long-term memory.

These are also addictive medications.

Steroids

Cortisone, Prednisone, and anything else ending with "-one" are the bad guys here. Steroids reduce inflammation using the body's stress response, and your brain experiences the same thing as when you are in the most stressful situation of your life, except that the chemicals (steroids) are even more intense than you body can naturally make itself. Steroids cause mental conditions requiring treatment in 20% of those who take them, and 75% of those people feel some mental alteration that is relieved when the drug is discontinued.[58]

Antibiotics

We already talked about the fact that antibiotics cause inflammation, which is a possible cause of dementia. But there's a particularly nasty class of antibiotics on the market called fluoroquinolones which deserve special attention. Avelox, Cipro, and Levaquin are the three most commonly prescribed, but you can identify them by the suffix "-floxacin."

Reactions of the central nervous system are common, with people self-reporting memory loss, psychosis, and other issues like pain, tingling/numbness, anxiety, dizziness, and more.[59] This is in addition to other common and/or severe reactions which have included gastrointestinal problems, tendon rupture, heart arrhythmia, and a whole mess of others.[60] The reason is because of the addition of a fluoride molecule, which helps the antibiotic permeate into hard-to-reach tissues.

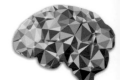

Unfortunately, that also increases permeability into the brain and spinal cord. And fluoride, as we've already discussed, is a known neurotoxin.

Generally speaking these antibiotics are only prescribed in special cases and/or as a last resort to kick infections that ordinary antibiotics can't reach. But that's not always the case, and even if it is there may be other options, so be wary if you get a prescription for one of these and ask if there are any other options available.[61]

Antihistamines

Dimetane, Vistaril, Benadryl, ChlorTrimeton, and Clistin are all antihistamines — and who would think something as common as an antihistamine could cause cognitive decline? Yet it does. Histamine is a neurotransmitter that the brain uses to cause wakefulness. We make it during the day to be awake and thinking. In local tissues it causes increased blood flow and itchiness like allergies and mosquito bites. In the stomach histamine is needed for stomach acid to digest food proteins and minerals, and defend us against bacteria, parasites, and fungi.

So antihistamines stop all those functions — including wakefulness and thinking. They also interfere with acetylcholine, the primary neurotransmitter for learning and memory.

Benzodiazepines

These drugs are prescribed for muscle spasms, seizure prevention, anxiety, irritability, and delirium. They calm you down. Sometimes benzodiazepines are prescribed for insomnia or depression. Xanax, Valium, Dalmane, Librium, Klonopin, Versed, Doral, Restoril, Halcion, and Ativan are in the first list of these drugs but also consider Centrax, Serax, Paxipam, Posom, Tranxene, and Librax.

Benzodiazepines cause memory loss by slowing down the activity in the brain that transfers information from short-term memory to long-term memory. This is why anesthesiologists use them -- so you won't remember how unpleasant surgery or any medical procedures are.

Benzodiazepines should only be used for short periods of time, especially if you are elderly. Chronic use of these drugs leads to memory impairment.[62] A 2014 study showed that if you took daily doses for 90 to 180 days, your chance of an Alzheimer's diagnosis rose 32%. If you took daily doses for more than 6 months, the risk increased 84 percent.[63] In fact, the study showed this strong association whether you took the 180 doses every day for 6 months, or spread it out over 5 years. It didn't matter. The people who took fewer than 90 doses had a much-reduced risk compared to the people taking benzos for longer.

Antiseizure Medications

You don't have to have epilepsy to be prescribed Phenytoin or Dilantin. You could have mood disorders, bipolar disease, nerve pain, or mania. Other examples of drugs in this category include Topamax, Depakote, Trileptal, Potiga, gabapentin (Neurontin), Diamox, Tegretol, Mysoline, Gabitril, Depakene, Zonegran, and Lyrica.

These drugs work by interfering with the central nervous system signals. This means you can't get the proper nerve flow, which in turn causes memory loss.[64]

Sleeping Pills

Ambien, Lunesta, and Sonata make you sleepy, which may be good to a point but when you have amnesia or can't remember where you are driving, it's less than ideal. These drugs interfere with your ability

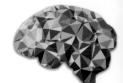

to remember new things, and while they do help you fall asleep a few minutes faster, they also stop you from remembering how hard it was to fall asleep or if you were sleeping poorly. These drugs have not been found to help with sleep maintenance (staying asleep), only sleep onset (falling asleep).[65] They are also addictive.[66]

Drugs for Incontinence

Overactive bladder is common in the elderly and it's treated with Enablex, Deltrol, Sanctura, Ditropan XL, Oxytrol, or Myrbetrig. These drugs work to stop acetylcholine from acting in the body, but learning and memory need acetylcholine.

What's the bottom line here? You'll have to decide for yourself but perhaps it's that just about any medication you could be prescribed has the potential to interfere with brain functions. Your brain is a victim of prescription medications. There must be natural alternatives for some of these that don't have these types of risks!

Chapter 4: When Should I Get Tested?

In a recent study, 2,125 people without dementia aged 65 or older took three tests:

a) the **East Boston Memory Test,** where the participant is told three sentences, each of which contains two ideas, and the participant has to immediately retell the story after hearing it;

b) the **Symbol Digit Modalities Test**, in which they paired numbers or letters with specific geometric figures; and

c) the **Mini Mental State Exam** which is commonly used to measure the progress of Alzheimer's.

The people who scored worst on those exams were much more likely to develop cognitive disorders like dementia decades later. The conclusion was that *the prodromal phase (the phase before disease symptoms are noticed) is very long for dementias.*[67]

This is good news (even if you think it isn't!) because it means that what you do now to protect your brain can impact you far into the future.

Normal vs Abnormal Memory Loss

We've all experienced that moment. You can't find your car keys or — perhaps for some of you who still know how to paint the town red — your car. You duck and run at church because you have passed the 6-month grace period for forgetting the pastor's wife's nickname and are slowly coming to the realization that you will have to find a new church just from sheer embarrassment. You just can't ever seem to remember things!

We all forget which kid we are talking to. We all lose our cell phones (and can I just give a plug to www.wheresmycellphone.com as my personal savior in that department?). We all have that moment where we look at the word "truck" — a word we have spelled successfully our entire adult lives — and come to the conclusion that "That's just not right. That is not how you spell truck." I knew a woman once who named her kids alphabetically and who would literally work her way from "A" on down until she saw the look of fear in the right kid's eyes and knew she had landed correctly.

These are not moments which should stir fear in our hearts. They are just moments. But they do beg a question: When should we panic? Exactly what kind of memory loss is "normal" and what is not?

There is a difference between mixing up your kid's names and not knowing your kids. Most people would have no trouble making that distinction. But what about the mushy middle? What are some signs that — taken in the right context — should generate a trip to the GP?

According to physicians at the Center for Brain-Mind Medicine at Brigham and Women's Hospital in Boston, there are many normal memory deficits which should NOT trigger any alarm.[68] These include:

- General absent-mindedness;
- A short-term block in recalling a memory;
- A tendency to forget events or facts over the course of time;
- Recalling something inaccurately, in part;
- Recalling something inaccurately, because of the power of suggestion; or

- Having a memory that is colored by mood, bias or experiences.

Generally, if you forget something but can recall it sometime afterwards, that's relatively normal.

Here are some other examples of what's considered "normal" memory issues:

- You might pause to remember certain directions, but you don't get lost in familiar places.
- You occasionally can't find the right word, but you have no problem holding a conversation, and you don't use words incorrectly, or repeat phrases and stories in the same conversation.
- You can recall incidents of forgetfulness and describe them, as opposed to remembering times when memory loss caused problems.
- You still have good judgement and decision-making abilities and don't make inappropriate choices.

Available Testing Options

No one seems to want to talk to their doctor about lapses in memory. Why is that? There seems to be a fear that talking about it will put flesh on the bones. But there are simple exams that can be performed by a physician (or even by a family member or by yourself) which can give quick guidance. And while early detection does not necessarily mean that cognitive decline can be stopped, it does give you information. And, best case scenario, you'll be able to stop worrying!

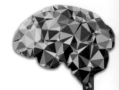

The SAGE Test

The Self-Administered Gerocognitive Exam (SAGE)[69] test is a quick exam you can take in the privacy of your own home. It's easily downloadable, can be completed in 15 minutes, and is great for determining whether or not you should seek out a more formal evaluation. The test items are things like "name the following pictures" or "draw this shape," and it tests classical executive function capabilities by asking the user to "path-find" using both sequential numbers and letters. Take this test at http://wexnermedical.osu.edu/patient-care/healthcare-services/brain-spine-neuro/memory-disorders/sage #SAGE%20Test

The Mini-Cog Test

The Mini-Cog with Functional Activities Questionnaire[70] is an even shorter test (3 minutes), designed to be administered by family members or peers, with a 74% accuracy rate for identifying mild cognitive impairments (MCI). MCI is sometimes seen as an early precursor to dementia. During this test, the user is asked to repeat the names of three items, draw a simple wall clock, and then repeat the words from the initial part of the test. Take this test at http://www.alzheimersreadingroom.com/2009/03/mini-cog-test-for-alzheimers-and.html

The Mini-Mental

If either of the previous two tests shows something suspicious, it's definitely time to have a talk with your doctor. There is a very simple, 8–10 minute screen which is the test of choice of many primary care doctors for memory. This screen, known as the Mini-Mental State Exam[71] has been in use for over 40 years and benefits from its quickness and longevity. However, the Mini-Mental does not test well for executive function, the loss of which is one of the first siren calls made by the brain. Executive function is necessary for organization, planning, and following a plan to meet a goal, and unfortunately, the Mini-Mental can miss early signs of decline in executive function. Take this test at http://www.alzheimers.org.uk/site/scripts/documents_ info.php?documentID=121

Montreal Cognitive Assessment

There is another test, known as the Montreal Cognitive Assessment[72] (MoCA), which seems to better tease out early cognitive decline. Both the Mini-Mental and the MoCA test orientation (time, date, and place) and both measure attention, concentration, language, memory, conceptual thinking, and the ability to calculate. But the Mini-Mental has trouble picking up early signals of decline that the MoCA is able to detect by making use of an executive function test (drawing lines from number to letter in correct order). The MoCA takes slightly longer to administer (10-12 minutes) and is less user-friendly for the administrator. Some doctors have taken to using both tests as a shotgun approach. Take this test at www.mocatest.org.

Conclusion

Fear can be paralyzing. But there is nothing to be gained by avoiding a simple test. Start with the SAGE or the Mini-Cog and see if something stands out, then make an appointment if it does. While these tests are not fool-proof, they do catch signs of early cognitive decline which might be ignored without formal testing.

Chapter 5: What Does Your Brain Need?

5.3 million. According to the Alzheimer's Association, that's how many of our nation's populace currently has Alzheimer's disease[73] — a shocking number by any measure.

But let's take a moment to think about brain health across the whole continuum. If brain health exists on a spectrum, with Alzheimer's and dementia lurking at one end, at the other is the "perfect brain," a state of *complete mental clarity* in which no one resides. But if there was a proven way to move just one tick closer towards that state of complete mental clarity, what would that mean to the Alzheimer's sufferer and to the rest of us?

It would mean remembering where we left the car keys. Or how to fill-out Wednesday's crossword puzzle. Or who that woman at church was (just in the nick of time before embarrassing ourselves).

Perhaps more importantly, it would mean knowing how many of the day's pills had already been consumed and — better, by far — why they were being consumed in the first place. It would mean the mental clarity to know that you needed to talk to your heart doctor about the pills your internist just put you on, because you can feel something isn't right and you have the cognitive wherewithal to associate those strange new physical symptoms with the new pink pill you started last week.

So how do we get there?

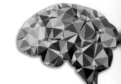

A Healthy Diet

We live in an age where there is no lack of advice on nutrition. Every television talk show host has an opinion and no two seem to agree. The truth is, no one knows *everything* about the relationship between the foods you choose and your brain power, but there are some facts that have stood the test of time.

You Have to Eat

Forget your body for a moment. Forget feeding your bones, your muscles, your blood and your organs. Pretend they are all working on auto-pilot. *You still have to eat*. The brain needs fuel and it needs it on a regular basis.

One of the strange quirks of moving through middle age and into later years is that, for some people, appetites diminish. You look at food and it doesn't seem to hold the same appeal. Food doesn't feel or taste the same in the mouth. (Did you know there is a whole industry out there devoted to getting people to like the "mouthfeel" of foods? If a food feels weird in our mouths, we won't eat!)

Sadly, for people with a diminished eating pleasure, this disinterest in food can become so radical, so profound that some people even enter a stage which doctors have taken to calling the "anorexia of aging." Recently, researchers have taken on the task of determining if this loss of appetite might be associated with the decline in neurocognitive performance seen in depressed adults. Their findings? Indeed, it is. Researchers found that late-onset depression is almost always coupled with cognitive decline, and that a loss in appetite might be a "marker" for the mental decline.[74]

Ah, that's not me, you protest, I eat like a horse! Even eating may not be
enough. As our bodies age, our gastrointestinal tracts do not function
as they did "in the old days". Our mouths don't produce quite enough
saliva to start the digestive process early, the food isn't mechanically
destroyed in our stomachs, or chemically broken down as completely, or
transported as quickly through our intestines (constipation, anyone?),
or absorbed into the walls of the intestines as readily. Frustratingly,
just about the time we settle into our retirement years, our guts start
to fail us, and the end result is less food for the brain, not to mention
almost every other organ system in the body (nervous, musculoskeletal,
cardiovascular, immune, and skin systems).[75]

This decline in the old GI tract means that not only do you have to eat, you
have to eat the *right* foods.

One last thing on this subject: Earlier I talked about how melatonin is
made from serotonin, and the resulting impact that has on sleep. Ninety-
nine percent of our serotonin is made outside of the nervous system in
our gut and other organs, which is why gut health is crucial for brain
health.[76] Eating well not only gives our brains a good supply of nutrients,
it helps our guts make plenty of serotonin (which is where 90% of
serotonin is made).

Fad Diets Come and Go for a Reason

Calories are not all created equal. If you don't believe me, try to live on
fast food for a month. Or lemons and organic maple syrup (a popular
"cleanse" diet). Or even energy bars. Take a moment to click through
Netflix for the latest documentary on some poor soul who got talked
into ruining his health so that the public could "see if it's possible to live
on the Big Mac alone." Fad diets come into vogue, usually supported by

some charismatic supporter on television or in the supermarket rags, and then they die a slow and largely unnoticed death.

We know the effect these fads have on our bodies. But what do such diets do to our brains? Nothing good. The typical Western diet (lots of bad fats and simple carbohydrates and sugar) has been linked with cognitive impairments. Researchers have come to believe that this kind of high sugar and bad fat diet can actually disrupt memory through altering the blood-brain barrier and creating dysfunction in the hippocampus,[77] which is more susceptible to physical stresses compared to other regions of the brain. Many parts of the brain can tolerate an onslaught from environmental toxins, or dramatic changes in the body's cardiopulmonary and metabolic states, but the hippocampus notices. And the hippocampus plays a very important role in memory and specific types of learning.

So, is a **low fat diet** the way to go? No. No, no, no! Low levels of dietary fat, coupled with high levels of dietary carbohydrates, produces a cascade of other problems. The brain is not able to function without fats. It is essential for our diet. It fills us up (provides satiety), stabilizes our blood sugar, gives us a consistent delivery of energy over time, keeps our brains supplied with necessary nutrients and fat, and helps us restore damaged blood vessels and cell membranes. This also doesn't mean that saturated fats are "bad" and unsaturated are "good." Your cell membranes are 50% saturated fat, so if you want you body to function, you have to eat good fats and not "fake" fats like hydrogenated fats or trans fats, especially along with a high carbohydrate diet. Not to mention that fat tastes good which goes a long way towards helping maintain any diet.

Interestingly, there is a huge body of research that supports the idea that the development of cognitive diseases, such as Alzheimer's, can be partially predicted by looking at diet. Alzheimer's disease, is being called by researchers "type 3 diabetes" where there is a strong connection between diet and onset.[78] Most people understand the relationship between eating too many poor-quality carbohydrates and developing insulin resistance. But the piece that most people don't understand is that insulin also serves a function in brain signaling.

In 2012, animal researchers looked at what would occur if they disrupted insulin's proper role as a neural signal. The result was something pretty much akin to dementia.[79] Many researchers are starting to speculate that the low-fat "doctor approved" diet trend that has swept the country for the last 40 years has been a terrible mistake, reducing the very macronutrient your brain has needed, and contributing to the escalating epidemic of Alzheimer's.

Energy for the Brain

While the body mainly relies on blood glucose to feed its cells, there are other sources of energy it can use, too. Ketones are an important one, typically made in the liver from fats and proteins, but recent research has discovered that the brain also makes its own ketones.[80]

We usually only make ketones when we don't have any carbohydrates in our diet, including when we are starving and just don't have any type of food at all. In 24 hours without carbohydrates the liver will start using ketones as fuel, and in a few days and weeks without carbs other organs will do this too. (This is how the Atkins diet works.)

The brain is the last organ to use the ketones made in the liver, and it takes about a month without carbohydrates to reach this point. But when it does start using these ketones, it becomes immune to the ups and downs that sugar caused in the past. The body can maintain a steady supply of ketones in the blood much more easily than a steady supply of glucose — a phenomenon that Johns Hopkins Hospital has been using to help children control epilepsy since the 1920s.[81] It probably works by

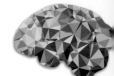

reducing the stress of low blood sugar on the brain, since low blood sugar can trigger seizures or migraines in people who are susceptible.

For developing babies, breast milk doesn't just contain sugars and immune cells, it also contains medium length saturated fats which the brain can use almost directly for fuel. Medium length saturated fats (also called medium chain triglycerides) are digested differently and faster than other fats, bypassing the lymphatic system and going directly to the liver.[82] They also don't need carnitine, a transporter molecule which other fats require to be shuttled into the mitochondria (the part of the cell that converts the fuel into energy). And the brain can convert medium chain triglycerides into useable ketones all by itself.[83]

Breast milk also contains an enzyme that allows babies to digest 100% of the cholesterol they eat. Cholesterol is usually quite difficult to digest, but plays a vital role in brain health in general (the brain contains 25% of the body's total cholesterol) and especially the developing brain of a baby.

When you remember that 87% of a baby's metabolism is used by its brain, and add in the fact that a baby has 2½ times the metabolic rate of an adult (at that rate a man weighing 170 pounds would need 7000 calories a day), you can start to appreciate just how much of a difference breast milk makes to a growing baby's brain.

For adults, there aren't a lot of foods in the Western diet that contain these medium length saturated fats, but butter, coconut oil, and palm kernel oil are a few of the places we can get them.

A Diet for Brain and Body

So what kind of diet *does* support brain health?

The obvious answer is the polar opposite of the dietary factors we talked about in Chapter 2. This means:

- Lots of vegetables;

- Healthy fats;

- Organic as much as possible;

- Meat, eggs, and dairy raised in as close to the animal's natural environment as possible (grass-fed cows, pasture-raised chickens, etc.);

- Low glycemic, low grain, low carb;

- NO processed foods; and

- NO sugar (or sugar substitutes), artificial sweeteners, preservatives, or other ingredients you don't recognize or have trouble pronouncing.

More specifically, there are a large number of studies currently underway investigating the effectiveness of certain foods on cognitive health. The National Institute on Aging is examining the benefits of omega-3 fatty acids, lipoic acid, blueberries, and coconut oil on brain function. Even walnuts, dark chocolate, avocados, and eggs are making a splash in the research.

OMEGA-3S have received a lot of air time for their spectacular effects on the heart, but they appear to be just as useful for reducing the effects of age on the brain. Omega-3s help with almost every role the brain must assume in its role as a repository for memory. Omega-3s help you retain facts and learned knowledge, they improve attention and they increase the ability to recognize people and objects. Omega-3s can be added to the diet by consuming fish, especially salmon or halibut, flaxseed oil (be very careful to keep it fresh), or dietary supplements.

COCONUT OIL has made a lot of headlines lately as the latest superfood to decrease the risks dementia associated with Alzheimer's. As one of those ketone foods we talked about above, there is some emerging research looking at the ability it has to improve the ability of the brain to function in insulin resistance. Although the research is preliminary, the National Institute of Aging has noticed and is now investigating its long-term use.

BLUEBERRIES are chock-full of antioxidants which help promote overall health, reduce inflammation and circulation, including obviously in the brain.

WALNUTS have been heralded as "anti-Alzheimer's" foods because of their chemical makeup including vitamins B and E, Omega-3s, and more.

EGGS (poor, demonized eggs!) are back and better than ever. For decades, the baby-boomer generation was warned against the inevitable onset of heart failure due to their morning eggs and bacon, but eggs have been vindicated in heart health and now are emerging as a great way to get choline, a necessary precursor for acetylcholine.

CHOCOLATE. Finally, a reason to eat chocolate without hiding your stash! Dark chocolate (85%) contains cocoa flavanols, which are antioxidants that circulate through the body, fighting free radicals and preventing cellular damage and decay. Dark chocolate has also been shown to enhance memory by protecting and supporting a special part of the brain known as the dentate gyrus.

Round out your diet with **avocados** for brain-healthy magnesium and you are well on the way to a "brain supportive" diet.

Regular Physical Activity

Exercise is a powerful way to improve health. Just like anything that reduces blood flow to the brain can increase your chances of dementia, anything that increases blood flow can slow or stop that process. It has been seen for decades, and is borne out in research, that physical exercise, whether it is gardening, walking, or being involved in sports, can significantly drop your chances cognitive decline.

It can treat depression when drugs alone are not working,[84] and in fact it is just as effective as Zoloft at treating depression with the added benefit of making people healthier.[85] Exercise stresses our bodies in a good way and causes positive adaptations. We add a little muscle, we become more insulin sensitive, we produce more repair hormones like human growth hormone and our organs become stronger to support the muscles.

Using your body causes the body's repair and maintenance systems to engage and keep us strong. Better circulation and more steady blood sugar are great things for brain health.

Also, lactic acid is a great fuel source for the brain. You may remember from school that anaerobic exercise is the kind where our muscles are forced to do work faster than oxygen can be delivered. When this happens, our muscles break down glucose into lactic acid.

Endurance athletes in particular know that if they use up too much blood sugar, they will effectively run out and become barely able to stay conscious, much less continue to exercise as intensely as they have been. They call this "bonking" or "hitting the wall," and anyone who's been there will tell you that it takes days to recover from.

What happens is over the next 2–3 days, the lactic acid gets circulated back to the liver to be built back up into glucose so that every organ can use it again.

But the brain still needs energy in order to survive. So it has specialized cells that can use lactic acid as a fuel for days after exercise.[86] This capability isn't powerful enough to prevent bonking on a 100-mile bicycle ride, but it does prevent us from passing out on that ride. Even better, when we do normal exercise like lifting weights, the lactic acid actually *improves* brain function. *The brain prefers lactic acid to glucose.*[87] It is like the high grade gasoline for performance cars.

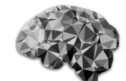

It's been shown that people with mild cognitive issues see improvement with consistent exercise.[88] The Honolulu-Asia Aging Study reported that men who walk at least 2 miles a day are 1.8 times less likely to develop dementia over a follow-up period of 6 years.[89]

Even if you have some health issues that might make exercise difficult, the exercise you *can* put in will make a difference. In people who have already had heart failure, "reductions in physical activity predicted acute decreases in attention/executive function in older adults with heart failure."[90]

And, of course, physical activity has the advantage of health benefits that are not confined to cognitive function alone, as suggested by research on depression, quality of life, falls, cardiovascular function, and disability.

Developing New Neural Pathways

Once upon a time it was thought that the adult brain was "fixed" and incapable of producing new neural pathways, but we now know better. The brain is capable of neurogenesis, especially in the hippocampus and cerebral ventricles, and, yes, exercise stimulates this growth.[91] In a way, physical activity signals cells to start acting like stem cells, capable of new growth. In addition, exercise increases the brain's "baseline activity" which also stimulates cellular growth.

But the brain doesn't need new growth in order to stimulate better cognition. The brain is incredibly underutilized, meaning we don't operate at anything close to max capacity. And that means that the brain can always find ways to overcome obstacles (like a stroke or brain injury or even the effects of aging) which life throws into its way.

The method by which this is done is called *plasticity*. When specific pathways in the brain are blocked or damaged, the brain can develop alternate pathways, circumventing those blockages. This also increases the brain's myelin sheathing, improving the brain's overall function by increasing the transmission speed of electrical impulses.

In their study of brain health, Cotman and his peers found that "exercise sets into motion an interactive cascade of growth factor that has the net effect of stimulating plasticity, enhancing cognitive function . . . [and] stimulating neurogenesis."[92]

Further research has found that there's no question exercise helps prevent and reverse cognitive decline. A recent study shows that regular exercise can stop brain shrinkage, even if you "have dementia in your genetic pool."[93] In one fascinating study, seniors in their 60s, 70s, and 80s who exercised at least three times a week, even with exercises that seem intellectually unstimulating like swimming, cycling, or walking, showed a dramatic increase in brain activity.

Other studies have shown that even those who have already developed symptoms of dementia can benefit from exercise to improve cognitive function and allow them to be better able to perform activities of daily living.

Weight Training

There are dozens, if not hundreds, of studies cited in systematic reviews (including those done by the Cochrane Collaboration, the gold standard of research) that support the idea that good old fashion, regular aerobic training have been shown to improve many aspects of cognitive function, e.g., memory, decision making, problem solving, and attention.[94] But what about other kinds of exercise? Does exercise have to be aerobic? Does it have to be regular?

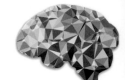

Resistance exercise has long been seen as the lowly stepsister of aerobic exercise. Well, it may not get invited to the ball, but it isn't sitting home crying over it! Specific resistance exercises have been found to combat cognitive decline among the senior set. Weight training, even as infrequently as once or twice a week, has been shown to improve executive function in seniors.[95]

We've mentioned executive functions before, but let's talk about them a bit more now. When you show the ability to selectively pay attention to the cashier at the bank (and ignore, or resist snapping at, the super-rude teenager on her iPhone next to you), you are resisting temptations and thinking before you act, practicing inhibitory control. Whenever you have an "aha!" moment where you think outside the box, you are practicing a cognitive flexibility. And when you show the capacity to hold information in your mind and manipulate it, you are practicing your working memory. All of these (and more) are executive functions, and they are our brains' core foundational elements of reasoning, planning, and creative problem solving.[96]

And the latest research supports that weight training, with machines or free weights, improves these functions.

But strength training doesn't just make you think faster. It may just make your day brighter. Exercising skeletal muscles help the body purge inflammatory chemicals associated with depression. These chemicals are naturally occurring in the body, but cause the brain stress and eventually damage. Muscles which are consistently exercised even show the ability to mobilize enzymes to join the fight against depression.[97]

Dual Task Training

As we just mentioned, the act of performing physical exercise can improve brain health. But all exercise is not created equally. Research has shown performing dual tasks (a cognitive task coupled with a physical task) may be just the ticket when working out to improve cognition. Instead of just "exercising", try to:

- Problem solve different ways to achieve movement. Ask "How can I get from here to there without standing up?" or "How can I make the least amount of noise?" and then explore all the different ways you can move.

- Have each activity you perform include a cognitive challenge as well as a physical one. (Try counting backwards by 3s or reciting directions from your garage to work while standing on one leg. It makes it ever so much harder!)

- Count exercises, multiply repetitions, recite while moving, and/or move different body parts in opposing directions.

- Use entrainment, which is a physical and cognitive trait often associated with perception of music; using entrainment, you move your body parts to the beat of the music or to a certain rhythm.

- Perform tasks that involve using both sides of the brain simultaneously, such as moving both arms in opposite directions at the same time, walking forward while moving arms to the side, or jumping up and down while moving arms to the side, alternating with forward and backward.

- Always push your boundaries. Begin with single-part tasks and then as mastery increases, gradually add parts to the sequence. Increase your speed gradually as quality and control of movement increases.[98]

No matter how beneficial exercise is, it does nothing if people do not want to do it. Instead of thinking of exercise as a limited category (swimming, running, walking, biking), it's time to start looking at a wider arena. Like to dance? Consider taking up salsa or a Zumba class.

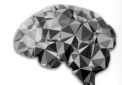

What about line dancing or New England contra dance, both dance styles where the entire room of people dance together. Do you enjoy martial arts? Then consider taking up Ai Chi, a form of martial arts performed in warm water. Or Yoga. The brain is wide-open to new possibilities, it just needs your body to take the lead.

Challenging Mental Activity

I'm not going to sugarcoat it here. Our brains, left unchallenged, do have a natural tendency towards decline with aging. What is *not* true is that the downward slope is inevitable. The brain retains plasticity, but it must be pushed around in order to tap into that inert neural flexibility. Think of your gray matter as a 3 lb. lump of malleable clay, awaiting the potter's hand. Memory, executive function, attention, and even the speed at which we process information are all fair game for training.

Great, but let's get down to brass tacks here. Exactly how does one go about molding a 3 lb. lump?

The answer is by **seeking out novelty in life**.

Physical therapists train balance in patients with injuries or diseases by pushing their patients to the edges of their current capacity — and then they push them over. That's one of the reasons that balance training works so well in the swimming pool. Because of the supportive and safe landing zone offered by the water, it is possible to push people repeatedly up to and over their existing balance thresholds. And that's how the body learns. It fails. It fails again. And then, one glorious day, it doesn't. It learns.[99] Eventually, the brain tells the body to grow bigger muscles, but in the meanwhile, the body learns to react quicker and to perform movements in a more logical manner.

Training the brain is really not much different from training the neuromuscular system. As long as individual continues to move through life in a straight line, never deviating from daily duties, never trying novel tasks, the brain never needs to adapt. But the newest research shows that the pursuit of challenging mental activity can enhance cognitive functions and take advantage of that quality of plasticity.[100] So what are some of the best options to pursue?

Play, Sing and Listen to Familiar Music

Music is different than almost any other form of language; it requires little in the way of mental processing, yet it evokes emotions and memories, some from days long gone by. When music is partnered with daily activities, such as chores, it can help individuals with dementia focus and successfully fall into a rhythm of normality. Even when the brain has fragmented to the point of severe dementia, the aptitude for performing musically and appreciating music remain. It's truly one of the last remaining abilities in even the most damaged of brains. Recently, some amazing science has emerged on the evocative power of music for even the most advanced Alzheimer's patients.[101]

But music is not just powerful for patients with Alzheimer's disease or other neurodegenerative disorders. Music evokes a powerful release of emotion in almost every human soul. It can lead to snapping fingers and dancing feet, to touch, to interconnectivity. And while listening to music activates the right side of the brain, singing brings the left side to life, creating a "whole brain" clarity that elevates mood, engages the spirit, and reduces stress and anxiety.

Every living person has a unique "favorite's list" but it's a safe bet that music played during formative times of life (early childhood, adolescence, young adulthood) will be linked to the greatest emotions.

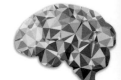

Go Back to School, Get a New Job . . . or Just Take Up Sudoku

Have you ever heard of the term *cognitive reserve?* If it makes you think of "putting a little away for a rainy day," you aren't far from the truth. Cognitive reserve is defined as the combined protective effect gained from a lifetime spent pursuing an education, an occupation, and meaningful cognitive leisure activities. It can be conceptualized as having something left in the tank at the end of the long road called life. Individuals who constantly work to gain new knowledge — whether that knowledge is nuclear physics or tie-dying — are putting reserves in the tank and it shows. In 2012, a huge study of over 13,000 people came to a simple conclusion: People who scored higher on "cognitive reserves" routinely showed a much lower risk of future cognitive impairment.[102]

Even something as simple as routinely playing number puzzles like Sudoku can make a big difference. These games are associated with spatial working memory, grammatical reasoning and episodic memory.[103] These three mental domains are strongly associated with the cognitive decline most often seen with aging, yet they are the very cognitive functions which blossom under training.

Engage in Computerized Cognitive Retraining

There is so much promise in the field of cognitive retraining that a whole industry is cropping up in support of the concept. Computer games like the Nintendo's **Brain Age** game[104] and online cognitive retraining services like **Lumosity** promise to stimulate the very fabric of your mental being. And interestingly, it appears that they do. There are more than twenty randomized clinical trials supporting the use of computerized training programs as a quick, often free, method to challenge and expand cognitive horizons.[105] Programs like Lumosity attempt to transform the science behind neurocognition into fun, "sticky" games which reinforce learning and memory. For example, they have taken a standard test called "go/no-go task" which was developed over a century ago to help psychologists evaluate the ability of people to control their impulses and they have converted this into a game called Robot Factory. By playing the game, the program is teaching you to tap into your executive functions and training your ability to make decisions.

Lumosity not your thing? Try a host of other brain-training apps, including:

- Brain Fitness Pro
- Brain Trainer Special
- CogniFit Brain Fitness
- Eidetic
- Fit Brains Trainer

Rich Social Interaction

We are a social people. Even the grumpiest curmudgeon amongst us has lived a life woven with rich social interactions. A study published in *Trends in Cognitive Science* says, "Humans, born to the longest period of abject dependency of any species and dependent on conspecifics across the lifespan to survive and prosper, do not fare well, whether they live solitary lives or they simply *perceive* they live in relative isolation."[106] Humans need interaction for physical health and for cognitive stimulation. Socialization is so important that physical isolation and loneliness can actually bring us to an early grave.[107] In fact, social interaction is such a dramatic factor that its very absence can be included

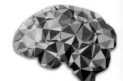

along with other more well documented risk factors for mortality, such as diabetes or high blood pressure.

But the lack of social networks does not just affect us physically; it may stunt our cognitive health as well. Look at the changes that are happening in traditionally socially interwoven societies, such as India. For thousands of years, the joint family has existed in India, often with multiple generations living under one roof. But this social network is showing signs of decay. The elderly population continues to grow while a low birth rate means there is not enough young family members to support them. But social norms are changing and the joint family is slowly dissolving. By studying this phenomenon, researchers were able to suggest a startling hypothesis: that the high degree of social engagement in India had served as a protective role against the onset of dementia and that this neuroprotective phenomenon was disappearing.[108] In other words, that the incidence of dementia is likely to increase merely because people no longer lived interwoven lives.[109]

Sleep and Rest

This is true for any area of your health, but it should be especially obvious for your brain that if you want to get better, you have to sleep.

Most of us understand intuitively that children sleep so much because they're growing. Having spent a full day working hard, sleep is the time when our children get that little bit taller and their organs get that little bit larger.

It's easy to forget that as adults we need the same thing — our organs have spent a full day working hard to keep the body running, and this is their opportunity to slow down and take care of themselves. This is when waste matter gets cleared from the brain,[110] it's when our immune, nervous, muscular, and skeletal systems recharge, it helps our wounds heal, and it has a ton of benefits related to mood, memory, learning, attention, and more.[111]

And yet, we spend our whole lives interrupting our natural sleep patterns through alarm clocks, caffeinated beverages, intense work schedules, and late night television.

And this doesn't just apply to night-time sleeping, by the way. Though culturally it's still not widely accepted in the U.S., there's a ton of evidence to support the fact that daytime naps improve moods, alertness, productivity, and memory, and the health benefits are now being proven too. Daytime naps reduce stress and blood pressure,[112] and siestas are associated with a 37% reduction in coronary mortality.[113] Anything that reduces blood pressure or heart disease will likely have similar effects on brain health.

Meditation or other forms of rest are also helpful. Memory consolidation (the actual conversion of short-term to long-term memories) happens when you're asleep,[114] but the evidence seems to suggest that it occurs during any period of prolonged restfulness.[115] Meditation is another opportunity to do that, and there's a ton of evidence that meditation has similar impacts as napping on cardiovascular and other measures of health. (And it might be more socially acceptable in your workplace to do on your lunch break.)

Smart Choices

There is no one pathway to a healthy brain, but there are so many dead-ends that can be avoided along the way. Immobility and isolation work hand-in-hand to make us into dullards. And a poor diet — for our stomachs and our brains — can drive us into cognitive decline or even an

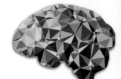

early grave. Simple choices are the answer, choices performed once, then again, and again, and so on and so on until inertia is overcome and the joy of it all overtakes resistance. That's all it takes. A few simple choices.

Chapter 6: Smart Supplementation

When Food is Not Enough

The typical American diet often fails to provide adults with the nutrients needed for health. Even individuals who take great pains to eat well — consuming no processed foods, little to no sugar, and only organic produce and pasture-raised meats — can do nothing about the fact that modern farming techniques have depleted the soil of many of the nutrients which have historically been part of our food chain. Crops are not rotated as they used to be. Modern fertilizers can force the ground to produce, but they cannot force the dirt to contain the same nutritional value as a properly rotated field could.

Additionally, American farms are often designed around the philosophy of "make everything taste better" and thus crops are grown with high fructose content, not nutritional value, as the primary goal. Consider the evolution of corn, a staple of the American diet:

> The wild ancestor of our present-day corn is a grassy plant called teosinte. It is hard to see the family resemblance. Teosinte is a bushy plant with short spikes of grain instead of ears, and each spike has only 5 to 12 kernels. The kernels are encased in shells so dense you'd need a hammer to crack them open. Once you extract the kernels, you wonder why you bothered. The dry tidbit of food is a lot of starch and little sugar. Teosinte has 10 times more protein than the corn we eat today, but it was not soft or sweet enough to tempt our ancestors.

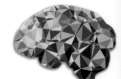

Over several thousand years, teosinte underwent several spontaneous mutations. Nature's rewriting of the genome freed the kernels of their cases and turned a spike of grain into a cob with kernels of many colors. Our ancestors decided that this transformed corn was tasty enough to plant in their gardens. By the 1400s, corn was central to the diet of people living throughout Mexico and the Americas.[116]

Many recent studies have pointed out that while children need more nutrients to grow, older individuals also need more nutrients to counterbalance the malabsorption associated with advancing age.[117] As humans get older, the GI tract performs its functions with less and less proficiency; compounding this effect is the fact that many medications commonly taken by baby boomers interfere with the absorption of nutrients.

So, it's clear that there *are* times when food alone is not enough. Because how much would you have to eat to make sure When the Europeans then began colonizing the Americas, they made note of the rich variety of colors — including red, blue, and green — associated with what we would now recognize as modern corn. But during the American Revolution they discovered the sweet yellow variety, which they then selectively bred over time into the supersweet white corn we mostly consume today — a variety that's orders of magnitude sweeter than the colorful varieties, and with a fraction of the nutrient density.

The degrees of separation between ancient teosinte and modern corn are many. And this is just one of countless examples of how our crops have changed to lose vital nutrients. Research has demonstrated that flash frozen fruits and vegetables are now often superior in nutrition to their fresh cousins,[118] because the fresh produce is picked too early (to allow it to be handled without bruising) and then shelved for days or even weeks before purchase. "Fresh" fruits and vegetables purchased at the grocery store (and shockingly, even at many farmers markets) have often been transported via non-refrigerated trucks, placed in warehouses, and shelved, waiting for your purchase, its nutritional value degrading with each passing hour.

The result: a tomato grown, harvested, and transported to market today will bear little nutritional resemblance to a tomato grown even a half a century ago. This is why we need supplements to support our health: to plug all the holes and to meet our basic nutrient needs.

But it's even more complicated than that.

You could make up for the deficiencies? Food is not enough for that pregnant women while her body is working to weave together her embryo's neural tube. And it's probably not enough for those who have hit menopause or their later years and who are on multiple medications.

But the good news is, the current state of evidence absolutely supports the use of supplements for cognition. Which means that very likely, the right supplements can make a positive impact on your brain health. They won't cure everything, but there is a lot to be excited about. Let's unpack the facts and find out more.

Essential Vitamins

There are 13 essential vitamins, called that because your body cannot make enough of them on its own, so you have to ingest (or inject) them. Those 13 essential vitamins are:

- Vitamin A
- Eight B Complex Vitamins
    - B1 – thiamin
    - B2 – riboflavin

- B3 – niacin
- B5 – pantothenic acid
- B6 – pyridoxine
- B7 – biotin
- B9 – folic acid
- B12 – cobalamins
- Vitamin C
- Vitamin D
- Vitamin E
- Vitamin K

Of these, **Vitamin D** and the **B vitamins** are often thought of as the "brain health" vitamins.

B Vitamins

B vitamins are crucial to our entire body's health, making it possible for us to extract energy from food, create red blood cells, and protect our nervous system. Consider the sad stories in the news about parents of newborns who found out the hard way that babies must get B vitamins or become ill.[119] Because vegetarians do not eat meat (and vegans do not eat any animal products), it is very difficult for babies of vegetarian parents to acquire B12 through breast milk or soy milk.[120,121], They need B Vitamin supplementation or they sicken. Period.

But it's not just babies (or pregnant women, or even post-menopausal women) who need supplementation. Clinicians have long been aware of the role that deficiencies in B vitamins can play on cognition, but the sum total of literature on the subject has skyrocketed since 2004.[122] As a result, B vitamin supplementation is fast becoming a standard for many populations.

The B vitamins all tend to work synergistically, serving as helpers to each other and to other essential vitamins, and because of that it is difficult to tease out discrete functions for each of them. Nevertheless, let's take a moment to examine what the four most well-researched B vitamins actually do for the brain and body:

Riboflavin (B2), is critical as a helper vitamin. It helps the body convert other B complex vitamins into a useable form, so without it vitamin B6 and folate (vitamin B9) would be next to useless. As just one example (a big one!), without riboflavin working in concert with the other Bs, it would be impossible for you to release energy from carbohydrates — without which, the brain and body would immediately begin to falter.

In addition to this crucial sidekick role, riboflavin acts on its own as an antioxidant working diligently to remove free radicals from the body.

Recently, higher dietary intake of riboflavin has been closely associated with better work recall and cognition. In a fascinating study, a team of researchers found that higher intake of B vitamins in early adulthood was associated with better cognitive function in late midlife.[123]

Like most B vitamins, riboflavin is water soluble, not fat soluble, which means that you cannot store it in your body for "whenever you need it." You must replenish your body's supply daily through diet or supplementation. Conventional wisdom has told us for years that it is difficult for people to be deficient in riboflavin, what with all the fortified foods available, but unfortunately, riboflavin is destroyed by light exposure, so fortified foods stored in clear glass containers (e.g., milk) get their riboflavin destroyed. What's more, foods rich in riboflavin but packed in water (e.g., canned vegetables), can lose

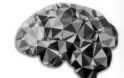

it through leaching into the packing water, which is then usually discarded during cooking or preparation.

A series of recent publications point to the possibility that up to 15% of the general population may have an inherited tendency toward a **secondary deficiency** in this B vitamin — meaning, they can eat a diet rich in riboflavin and still be deficient. This is due to a 1-2 combination punch created by a reduced ability to absorb the vitamin coupled with a greater tendency to excrete it in the urine. This unfortunate combination then seems to produces a homocysteine imbalance in the central nervous system. If this research bears out, riboflavin deficiency may actually emerge as "the most prevalent genetic risk factor" for terrible neurological diseases such as Parkinson's and dementia.[124]

Vitamin B6 is another of the essential B complex vitamins. And while B6 deficiency is rare outside of chronic alcoholism and frank malnutrition, B6 *insufficiency* is not. Why does this matter? Vitamin B6 works synergistically with folate to help it stimulate revascularization of the arteries leading to the heart. For a long while, folate has received all the credit, but recent research seems to show that, but for the presence of B6, folate would play no significant role in coronary revascularization.

So, you might be asking, that's all well and good, but what does revascularization of the heart have to do with the brain health? Glad you asked. The short answer is — a lot. Scientists studying cardiovascular disease have long believed in something called the **homocysteine theory** of cardiovascular disease.[125] Homocysteine is an α-amino acid that is produced when proteins begin to breakdown. Elevated homocysteine levels are considered potentially dangerous because it can damage arterial walls in the heart.

But this theory is not restricted to the heart anymore. Study after recent study has pointed out that the homocysteine theory can be applied equally well to vascular dementia and Alzheimer's patients.[126,127] Some researchers believe that too-high homocysteine levels cause mental impairments directly: in other words that elevated homocysteine acts as a toxin or poison of sorts.

Either way, the problem is the same. Elevated homocysteine levels affect cognitive health in a huge variety of ways, and vitamin B6 can be one piece of the solution for lowering them. As just a few examples, here are some of the results associated with lowering high homocysteine levels in the body:

- A slowing of the atrophy of the brain associated with aging;
- Enhanced cognition;
- Enhanced episodic memory (your memory of your own personal experiences);
- Enhanced semantic memory (your ability to remember things taught to you).

Folate (as folic acid) and Vitamin B12. Folic acid has many positive benefits including the ability to support cognitive processing speed, memory and fluency in healthy adults.[128] On the other end of the mental health spectrum, deficiencies have been shown to play a significant role in neurodevelopmental disorders, psychiatric disease, and dementia.[129]

Let's think about this for a minute. When scientists want to test for the benefits of vitamin B supplementation, it is very useful to have a population of people who intentionally abstain from eating foods that are rich in that vitamin. In India, a country with a high population of vegetarians, many people suffer from low vitamin B12 status and high homocysteine levels; in other words, they are the perfect population to investigate the effects of vitamin B12 supplementation! One such study investigated whether individuals could lower their homocysteine levels more by eating lots of green leafy vegetables or by taking a Vitamin

B12 supplement.[130] The people who ate cooked green leafy vegetables showed no improvement in vitamin B12 levels, and their homocysteine levels failed to drop. Those who took the supplements showed higher B12 levels and a significant drop in their high plasma total homocysteine concentrations. Of course, this is not surprising because B12 is found in animal products, not in plants, which is why it's a common deficiency in vegetarians.

Folate, on the other hand, *is* found in vegetables. In fact, that's where the word comes from — *folia* in Latin, meaning leaves or foliage — and folate is also key in keeping homocysteine levels down. In fact, one of the findings in a recent gold-standard systematic review was that longer-term supplementation with folic acid and Vitamin B12 appeared to improve the cognitive function of healthy older people with high homocysteine levels.[131] The review also supported the idea that folic acid could improve the response of people with Alzheimer's disease to some of their medications. Greater vitamin B12 intake has even been associated with a higher volume of gray matter in the brain,[132,133] and in people who already have mild cognitive decline, taking folic acid, B6, and B12 can slow the rate of brain atrophy.[134]

Clearly, the B vitamins play a huge role in mental health!

Vitamin D

Vitamin D, often called the sunshine vitamin, is mainly produced by our skin during exposure to sunlight. You'd think that would mean that there was little to no risk of deficiency in this vitamin, but the overzealous use of sunblock and avoidance of direct sunlight has created an unintended consequence of low Vitamin D levels, especially for people who live in northern climates. The now-debunked low-fat recommendations contributed to this, too, as vitamin D is fat soluble and needs the fat in foods to be absorbed. Vitamin D insufficiency and deficiency are now both considered major potential problems for many adults.

Supplementation with Vitamin D is considered standard practice for fall prevention in the at-risk baby boomer generation. Vitamin D is also responsible for helping manage the calcium levels in the body and it is a crucial factor in the ability for the body's cells to communicate with each other.

But what about Vitamin D's role in mental function? According to the Vitamin D Council, lower vitamin D blood levels are linked to a higher risk of cognitive impairment.[135] This has been confirmed in many studies summarized on their site, including:

- Adults with low vitamin D blood levels performed much worse on a cognitive performance test.[136,137]

- Men with lower vitamin D levels performed worse on a test with numbers.[138,139]

- Adults aged 65 years and older with vitamin D levels less than 12 ng/ mL were 2.3 times as likely to have cognitive impairment as those with vitamin D levels above 26 ng/mL.[140,141]

- Older adults with vitamin D levels below 10 ng/mL had a 60% increased risk of decline in global cognitive function compared to those with vitamin D levels above 20 ng/mL. There was also a 30% increased risk of decline in decision making.[142,143]

- Adults greater than 65 years of age with vitamin D levels below 10 ng/mL had 4 times the increased risk of cognitive impairment compared to those with levels above 30 ng/mL.[144]

To get a big picture of what Vitamin D does, it helps to look to published systematic reviews. A 2013 systematic review showed that individuals with hypovitaminosis D (a fancy way to say a low level of vitamin D) display many negative cognitive consequences, for example a higher frequency of dementia or a tendency to score worse on cognitive tests.[145] Vitamin D deficiency has also been shown to play a not-fully-understood role in depression.[146] Individuals with depression are routinely found to have lower vitamin D levels; in fact, the lower the vitamin levels, the greater the odds for a depression diagnosis. Obviously, the ability to maintain adequate levels of Vitamin D is a vital part of brain health.

Since Vitamin D is fat soluble, unlike the B vitamins it can be stored in body fat for later use, so there is the possibility of overdoing Vitamin D intake if the nutritional supplement chosen is not balanced.

Fish Oil

For decades, fish has been described as brain food, and for good reason. Humans can manufacture many of the fats we need from other fats or from building blocks found circulating in the body. But this is not the case for omega-3 fatty acids. Omega-3s are essential fats — which, just like essential vitamins, cannot be made by the body so must be taken in by food or supplementation.

Certain kinds of nuts (especially walnuts), flax seeds, vegetable oils, and leafy vegetables are high in omega-3s, but the best way to get them is to eat fish — especially oily fish, like salmon, albacore tuna, sardines, mackerel, herring, and lake trout.

So what makes Omega-3s so very special? Without them, your cell membranes would leak and malfunction. You could not make certain hormones responsible for the gamut of your body's regulations (blood clotting, inflammation control, and so on). Without Omega-3s, you couldn't even contract or relax your arteries. Omega-3s play protective roles, helping the body to control autoimmune diseases like lupus and rheumatoid arthritis. They even bind to receptors in cells that are responsible for your very genetic code, your DNA.

And then there's the impact it has on your brain. In a 2015 study, researchers investigated whether the use of fish oil supplements would reduce cognitive decline and brain atrophy.[39] During a community initiative called the Alzheimer's Disease Neuroimaging Initiative, they used MRIs to examine the brain images of almost 500 people about two-fifths of whom had a diagnosis of Alzheimer's, while the rest did not. At the end of the study, they found that after taking fish oil supplements, those with normal cognition showed improved thinking and fewer signs of cognitive impairment. The use of fish oil even reduced the level of atrophy present in one (or more!) areas of the brain.

But, omega-3s aren't just known for their ability to slow cognitive decline of aging. They have also been heralded as a safer alternative to antidepressants. Antidepressants continue to hit the news cycle with story after story about side effects, including greater risk of depression and, of all things, suicide! Because of this, physicians and researchers are turning their eyes towards the potential benefits of more natural options — including use of omega-3 fatty acids.

Several studies have found that individuals taking antidepressants may show a reduction in sleep and sexual dysfunction, anxiety, and depression by adding omega-3s to their treatment plan.[147,148]

A huge scientific study of nearly 22,000 Norwegians investigated the role of fish oil on depression and helped answer whether or not fish oil could reduce the signs of depression.[149] In this study, the researchers compared those who took cod liver oil to those who did not. They also compared those who took it for the short-term to those who took it for a longer duration. Their results were fascinating. They found that those who took cod liver oil, especially those who took it for a longer duration, had significantly lower risk of depression. In fact, those who took the oil were

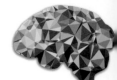

about 30% less likely to show clinical signs of this mood disorder. Just one more reason to consume omega-3s!

Essential Minerals

Vitamins are not the only game in town when it comes to brain health; certain minerals have a place at the table as well. Copper and zinc are two trace — but essential — minerals which have been shown to be important for cognition.

Copper

Copper, coupled with iron, is necessary for the body to form red blood cells. It also plays a role in preventing bone defects and producing healthy connective tissue. This mineral can be found in many types of foods, especially seafood, nuts and seeds, grain products, wheat bran cereal, and especially organ meats.

For the most part, copper is stored in the body within the bones and muscles, and the liver regulates how much can be found in the bloodstream at any one time. Copper deficiency can cause anemia and neural symptoms.[150] And while a copper deficiency may be a potential reason for impaired cognition, deficiencies in copper are rare unless zinc supplementation is being used.[151] Which brings us to …

Zinc

Zinc has a hypercritical role in the brain, so much so that a deficit in zinc can cause death of neurons. Zinc regulates the communication between the hippocampus and the brain's neurons, playing a direct role in improving learning capacity and memory, and so it appears that the right intake of zinc is a key part of achieving a "brain shield."[152] A 2013 systematic review confirmed this, showing that there is a positive association between zinc supplementation and improvement in cognition (though the authors stressed that this association needs to be investigated further before too many claims can be made).[153]

But while zinc clearly plays a critical role, more zinc isn't always better. Too high of a dosage of zinc can produce neurological problems, such as ataxia (a movement disorder), tingling in the fingers, and nerve pain in the limbs. Interestingly, these neurological symptoms are not produced by the presence of zinc itself, but because too much zinc can produce a copper deficiency.[154]

To better picture this, imagine the mineral see-saw going down on one side only to pop up on the other. The presence of the right amount of zinc keeps copper in check and reduces the possibility of copper toxicity,[155] but too much zinc can make copper levels too low. So just check to be sure that your zinc supplement comes with copper as well.

Iodine and Trace Minerals

Seaweed is your best source of iodine and it can help you kick out lots of toxic chemicals (fluorine, bromine, chlorine) and heavy metals (lead, cadmium and mercury). It is the definition of a superfood and historically was eaten by every human population that could trade with the coastal peoples.

It is mainly the iodine in seaweed that helps us do all of that. It also has compounds like algin that help us with heavy metal detoxification and is one of the richest sources of trace minerals as it has every single one! Trace minerals are needed for numerous enzymes in our brain and body. It's hard to get enough of these in our diet and there are so many that it's hard to put them all in a supplement. So add seaweed to your diet!

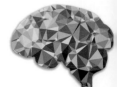

Amino Acids and Antioxidants

L-Theanine

Other than water, the world's most popular beverage is tea. Tea contains a special amino acid known as L-Theanine that can alter the brain's alertness and restfulness.

Have you ever known someone who operates well under pressure, someone who does not seem to experience any anxiety, even under stressful situations? Many people who do well under stress are exhibiting some of the benefits of tea consumption.

L-Theanine consumers can exist in a state of wakeful relaxation without ever feeling drowsy or falling asleep,[156] and are able to sustain their attention for longer periods of time when asked to perform difficult tasks, as evidenced by enhancement to the alpha-band activity of the brain.[157]

Tyrosine (N-acetyl L-tyrosine)

Tyrosine is an amino acid which functions as a chemical building-block of dopamine. N-Acetyl L-Tyrosine is a more heat-stable and soluble form of Tyrosine, which is often used in supplements.

The use of N-acetyl L-tyrosine as a supplement has grown in popularity very rapidly over the last decade. Its supporters claim that it does everything from helping to build muscle mass to helping to stimulate the brain by balancing neurotransmitter levels.

An interesting study to confirm this involved placing test subjects in "acute environmental stress" (or, in layman's terms, unbelievably cold water). The study verified that exposure to cold dampens mental performance (no surprises there!) and that supplementation with tyrosine protected working memory under that environmental stress.[158,159]

L-Carnitine (Acetyl-L-carnitine)

L-carnitine is a derivative of the amino acid lysine, and acetyl-L-carnitine is a very well-researched supplement synthesized from L-carnitine to be more biologically available.

For many years, acetyl-L-carnitine was considered an interesting biological curiosity with little to no practical application,[160] but this is no longer the case. Acetyl-L-carnitine (often referred to as ALCAR) is now a blazing hot subject matter in research, especially in the field of dementia and Alzheimer's research.

So what, exactly, is ALCAR?

It is believed that ALCAR serves as a powerful antioxidant by promoting the creation of a certain kind of free radical "scavengers" that roams the body. ALCAR supplementation has been used successfully to promote attention concentration, better reaction times, and improved performance on memory tests.

It is believed that ALCAR boosts the body's energy production at the cellular level (inside the mitochondria) and thus reduce both physical and mental fatigue.[161]

Studies have shown that daily supplementation with ALCAR can serve a protective function for the central nervous system; in fact, supplementation is showing great promise as a treatment for Alzheimer's disease, Down's syndrome, and Parkinson's.[162,163,164] Supplementation seems to provide the most dramatic results in patients with earlier onset or faster rate of decline of CNS disorders.

CoQ10

CoQ10 is shorthand talk for coenzyme Q10, an antioxidant made by the human body that's essential for all the basic functions of the body's cells. As humans age, our levels of CoQ10 decline and some of the results of this decline are what people think of as "getting old." Individuals suffering from medical conditions such as Parkinson's disease, cancer, diabetes, and heart disease have low levels of this important antioxidant.[165] CoQ10 also drops (sometimes alarmingly) with the consumption of statins and anti-hypertensive drugs, which are commonly taken taken by seniors.[166]

Fortunately, it is possible to increase the body's storehouse of this antioxidant by supplementing with a man-made version of CoQ10.

CoQ10 has been linked to so many wonderful benefits that it is hard to make a short list, but let's take a moment to hit some of the highlights. First, CoQ10 supplementation has been used to reduce high blood pressure and heart failure; in fact, the evidence for both of these conditions is particularly strong.[167] It has also been used to reduce the effects of high cholesterol, eye disease, asthma, and chronic fatigue. Some preliminary studies suggests that the use of CoQ10 coupled with other antioxidants and minerals may reduce the appearance of aging such as skin roughness and wrinkles.[168] Other research even suggests that a combination of CoQ10, acetyl-L-carnitine, and omega-3 may reduce the effects of age-related macular degeneration.[169]

But the most interesting and cutting-edge use of the man-made version of CoQ10 seems to be associated with its use to combat the effects of Alzheimer's disease, especially if used in the early stages. It all has to do with its ability to slow the rate of neuronal (brain cell) death. In the initial stage of Alzheimer's disease, scientists have discovered that there is a decline in the levels of energy metabolism; the cells are just not pumping out enough energy to take care of basic housekeeping. This appears to be due to damage in DNA at the mitochondrial level. Take a moment and think back to high school biology class. The mitochondria are the powerplants of the cells. If the cell's mitochondria are off their game, the amount of energy that they can produce just plummets. And while the pathophysiology of Alzheimer's is not completely known, we do know that this failure to produce energy, coupled with a decline in activity of something called the **electron transport chain**, may result in what we see as dementia.

The electron transport chain is the final stage in energy production; this is the process that leads to the formation of ATP (energy) in the mitochondria. To simplify the concept, think of what happens when you plug in a lamp. When the switch is turned on, it creates a chain reaction: electricity begins to flow, and it does so because one atom is stealing an electron from the atom next to it. This process continues again and again, with electrons "flowing" until the switch is turned off or the plug is pulled. The same process occurs in the brain. The electron transport chain is a long chain of compounds in which electrons are stolen and accepted. In short, it is an essential stage in the creation of energy . . . and without it, the brain slows down.

Supplementation with antioxidants appears to be quite useful for individuals who are suffering from cognitive challenges. Researchers have combined multiple supplements (including Omega-3s, selenium and certain vitamins) in an attempt to provide a counterbalancing effect, producing a moderate improvement in symptoms of dementia. This new and exciting area of research is known as **mitochondrial medicine** and it is focused at keeping the mitochondria with their (figurative) noses to the grindstone, doing the single greatest work of these powerhouses: producing energy.[170]

The end result of supplementation is an exciting glimpse into what can happen with prevention. If mitochondrial medicine, such as occurs with supplementation with CoQ10, is used early in the Alzheimer's game, it appears to be possible to produce a slowdown in the death of nerve cells in the brain.[171]

Herbal Support

There are many herbs that have been used for centuries to improve sharpness and memory, and recent research has started delving into the actions of these plants. The challenge is that plants are very complicated, and it's often not simply one compound in the plant, but rather the interaction of multiple compounds. Let's take a look at what are the most popular brain herbs.

Ginkgo Biloba

Ginkgo biloba is the rising star out of all the "memory boosters" currently being investigated. Physicians from European countries already routinely prescribe gingko for patients with dementia, and several systematic reviews have shown that ginkgo is at least as beneficial for management of dementia as the most common prescription medicines. Ginkgo biloba's strongest suit is its ability to improve blood flow in the small vessels of the brain (and elsewhere). But that is not the only effect of this wonder plant; ginkgo has also been shown to support:

- mental accuracy,
- mental calmness,
- short-term memory,
- general intelligence,

- visuospatial abilities, and
- attentional processing speed.

Ginkgo has even been shown to improve the ability to remember appointments, a well-known problem directly associated with middle-age.[172]

In 2015, researchers published a meta-analysis supporting the mental benefits of supplementation with ginkgo biloba.[173] First and foremost, they showed that ginkgo was both safe and well tolerated at many different dosages, although 120–240 mg were the most common dosages tested (and the amount that seemed to make the most difference). Second, according to some very large studies discussed in the analysis, ginkgo was shown to both slow and stabilize mental decline in patients with dementia or other cognitive impairments. But that's not all. The authors also touted the clinical benefits of ginkgo in many other related categories, including behavior, functional status, and global clinical change. Of special import is that fact that these positive results were seen with patients with Alzheimer's and dementia, yes, but also with patients with "mild" cognitive impairments.

An important note — you have to take ginkgo for a long-enough period of time, typically at least three months, to get the benefit. So if you decide to take it, make sure you stay consistent!

Ashwagandha Root

Ashwagandha root extract is a commonly used herb in Ayurvedic medicine. For hundreds of years, Ashwaganda root has been revered in Asia for its antioxidant, rejuvenating, and anti-inflammatory properties, but recent studies have shown there is more to love about this lowly root than its ability to protect the human body against cellular damage. Recent research has demonstrated that an extract from the root can be used to benefit the cardiopulmonary, endocrine, and central nervous systems. As just one example, Ashwagandha has been used clinically to help fight insomnia at night and anxiety by day.[174]

Ashwagandha root extract has even made the news as a possible way to tackle depression. In one compelling study, a group of adults given a high-concentration dose of Ashwagandha root extract for just sixty days showed startling results: they had substantially reduced levels of serum cortisol (which is one way to measure for stress and anxiety), were significantly less anxious and they slept better and longer at night, all with little to no negative side effects.[175]

Bacopa

Bacopa *(B. monnieri)* is another herb that has been shown to improve cognitive function. It has been used traditionally in Ayurvedic medicine for centuries for cognition and improving intelligence. In one study, test subjects over the of 65 showed significantly improved delayed word recall, could remember items and pick out important details amidst irrelevant information (the Stroop test), and as an added bonus, depression and anxiety decreased significantly as well.[176] Another study found the same results — that taking Bacopa for more than 3 months, at a dosage of 300 mg per day, significantly improved cognitive function and working memory accuracy.[177]

A rat study found that combining ginkgo and Bacopa had even better effects. The researchers could induce Alzheimer's disease in the rats with certain drugs and saw that not only did the rats have better memory in water maze tests, but that the herb combination was protective against a reduction in neurons and cholinergic neuronal densities (how Alzheimer's disease looks in the brain).[178]

Chapter 7: The 28-Day Plan

With everything involved in brain health, it unfortunately takes more than just a miracle pill to completely turn things around. That being the case, we've put together a 28-day plan, with one new element to introduce per week, which can have a significant impact. Reread the introduction if you want some motivation for taking these actions on, because these are the foundations to improving your brain function and preventing the specter of Alzheimer's and dementia.

There are more than four elements here, so we'll emphasize which ones are vital and which ones you can choose from. And just like any program, it's the constantly "getting back in the saddle" and practicing that makes this transform from new, unfamiliar actions to just what you do to take care of yourself.

Obviously, some of these involve more education and structure and we've provided what we can for those sections.

Strategy #1: Manage Your Blood Sugar VITAL

There's no doubt that Alzheimer's disease and dementia are driven in large part by sugar intake. We live longer now than in the past, which may be part of the reason that we see more cognitive decline, but we have also radically changed how we eat, and the biggest change is in how much sugar we ingest.

If you are worried about cognitive decline (and I would assume you are, since you're reading this book), you cannot get off sugar fast enough or completely enough. It is *that* bad for you. Never mind how it increases heart disease, or causes depression, or inflammation, or wrecks your

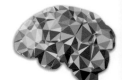

sleep. We're just dealing with your brain here, but if you take this on, the impact for your entire health will be enormous.

Sugar doesn't necessarily mean just candy or cookies. It also means refined carbohydrates like pasta and breads, which turn into sugar. It means the added sugar in most store-bought foods — everything from salad dressings to pasta sauce to ketchup to guacamole in a jar. It has tricky names, like corn syrup, or high fructose corn syrup, or dextrose, maltose, or anything with an -ose ending. And don't fall for the trick that just because it's organic it's better, or that brown sugar is better, or that maple syrup or honey or agave nectar are preferable (they're not), or that "heart healthy" or "whole grain" or "natural" mean anything.

If you are buying food items in bags, boxes or cans, more often than not, those foods will include some form of sugar.

As you can imagine, sugar is highly addictive, so for most people "just cut it out" is much easier said than done. For that reason, we have a whole program that's all about managing blood sugar (http://smartbloodsugar.com/). However, here's the summary of what it takes to make the changes necessary for your brain (this is also in one of the bonus materials):

1. Eat every three hours, or before you're hungry. This prevents sugar cravings.
2. Eat fat with everything. No exceptions. Fat provides the satiety response, and when your body is burning fat as fuel it helps keep your blood sugar levels stable.
3. Limit your carb intake. I'll give you two options for doing this:
   a. Max 100 grams of carbs per day, **or**
   b. Max 60 grams of carbs per day **not including green vegetables, carrots, or beets.**

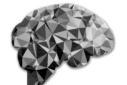

Most people find it too tedious to count every single carb for every single vegetable, which is why I offer the second option. Nobody got diabetes or Alzheimer's because they ate too many vegetables, so if you go to 105 or 110 grams of carbs per day it's not that big a deal, as long as those carbs are coming from nutrient-dense foods rather than from pasta or candy or sugared drinks.

The blood sugar management cheat sheet included in the bonus materials says what to count, but if you want the super condensed cheat sheet version, here it is:

- If it comes from anywhere other than the produce section in the grocery store, count it. This should be easy, because everything outside of the produce section comes with the nutrition information already on the label.
- Count colorful vegetables (except carrots or beets), including potatoes, sweet potatoes, corn, and beans.

And that's it. You don't have to count like this forever - after a month you'll have a pretty good idea of what you can and can't eat to get to 60 grams a day, but this will get you there in the meantime.

While this might sound a little daunting, it's not as hard as you think. You'll know you're on the right track when you start to notice that your moods, your energy, and your ability to concentrate are no longer as dependent on how recently you ate. You'll probably notice this improvement within a week, and while this won't necessarily immediately translate into better brain health, it definitely will over time.

You don't have to get this perfect, but if you were going to start somewhere, it would be here.

Strategy #2: Trade Real Food for Fake Food VITAL

You've heard it your whole life that you should eat fresh fruits and vegetables, or that "real" food is better than fake food. And you've heard that for a reason. Fake foods wreak havoc on your gut, your brain, and your health in general, and the more of them you eat the worse it gets.

What's fake food? Something processed and heavily marketed, filled with ingredients you wouldn't find in your own kitchen. Like frozen dinners. Frozen waffles. "Dessert" yogurts (as we call them) — have you seen the ingredient list on those? Things that come with a mix, like macaroni and "cheese" that's powdered, or something in an envelope to add flavoring to meat. Or how about American cheese "food", or cheese out of a can? What about butter alternatives? Those aren't real! Entire aisles of crazy drinks, chips and snacks, even low-fat food — as we often say to patients, did that low-fat milk come out of the cow that way? None of that is real food.

We like to tell people, if your grandmother wouldn't recognize what you're eating, it's probably not real food.

To feed your brain, you need food that actually has nutrition in it, and that stuff does not. If you want to reverse the damage that has happened so far (and we all have some), the highest quality of food you can afford will help. This looks like:

- As close to natural or organic or free-range meat, eggs, and dairy as you can find.
- Organic fruits and vegetables as often as you can. (Remember the soil quality issue? Organic vegetables are grown in much higher quality soil.)

- Foods that haven't been processed, changed, added to or subtracted from.
- Restricting how often you eat in restaurants (even the highest quality restaurants serve food that's processed).
- Learning how to make meals with these original ingredients.

We know this is the part that people tend to resist (along with the getting rid of sugar). We totally understand, and you don't have to do it all at once. But we ask you to consider this: you are reading this book because you either had some cognitive decline, or you're worried about it. When do you want to start?

The easiest place to start is at home. Peer pressure is powerful, and we know how hard it is to avoid cake at that birthday party, or ordering a pasta dish when you're at a restaurant. So the first place to cut it out is at home. If you just don't buy those things when you're at the grocery store, it quickly becomes much easier to avoid eating them.

The common suggestion here is to "shop the perimeter" of the grocery store. If you've never heard that term before, here's what it means: Most grocery stores (large ones in particular) are designed with produce near the entrance and their fresh meat and dairy along the outside walls. In the middle are all the shelf-stable items (stuff in bags, boxes and cans), which are full of preservatives, sugar, and artificial ingredients. By sticking to the perimeter of the grocery store, you'll get much more real food and avoid the fake stuff.

Start dealing with your food in pieces and parts. The first part is to reduce your refined carb and sugar intake (mentioned above), and this part might look like:

- Boiling some eggs and having them ready in the refrigerator
- Making tuna salad, adding some chopped celery, and eating that on a bed of lettuce or spinach (or both!).
- Switching that out with making chicken salad, or egg salad.
- Keeping some cut veggies on hand with hummus as a snack
- Eating some of your favorite raw nuts (just don't go crazy with the nuts!)
- Replacing the sugar you add to tea or coffee with stevia or xylitol, both of which are from natural sources
- Reducing your juice intake by watering it down, or replacing it completely with sparkling water
- Same thing with soda — replace it with sparkling water (they have flavored sparkling water, too!)

One neat way to get better at making food is to pick an ingredient you know nothing about (let's take the example of Swiss chard) and look up a recipe on the computer. Try doing this for a new meal or new ingredient once a week. As we tell our patients, someone, somewhere on the Internet, has solved your problem!

Strategy #3: Add Coconut Oil into Your Diet

We're just beginning to come out of the low-fat craze (talk about something your grandmother wouldn't recognize!), and now there's begun to be research in the specific effects of medium chain triglycerides, most often seen as coconut oil. As we mentioned before, coconut oil can help feed the brain, especially where there's insulin resistance.

While there have been plenty of animal trials that have shown that using medium chain triglycerides can be helpful for dementia, there have recently been human studies that have showed the same thing, including in Alzheimer's patients.[179] A 2004 study showed that administering β-hydroxybutyrate (which comes from ingesting medium chain triglyceride oils) turned around Alzheimer's disease in patients,[180] and another study that same year showed that you could reverse that improvement if you ate high carbohydrate:[181]

When a patient is treated for epilepsy with the ketogenic diet, a high carbohydrate meal can rapidly reverse the anti-seizure effect of the diet. It is therefore of interest that high carbohydrate intake worsens cognitive performance and behavior in patients with Alzheimer's disease.[182]

Research has shown variations in how much you need but at the moment it looks like the more you can do, the better. There was a case study of a woman who treated her husband's Alzheimer's with 5 tablespoons a day. One study saw an improvement just in one dose![183]

Of everything in this chapter, this is probably the easiest strategy to implement. Coconut oil comes in two forms, unrefined (also known as "virgin" or "raw") and refined. The refined in this case only means that the coconut proteins have been removed, which reduces or eliminates the taste of coconut, which can be helpful for some people. But other than that, the health benefits are the same. It tends to be solid under temperatures of 76 degrees, but you can buy it in a liquid form (MCT oil), if you'd like to add it to smoothies. Some of our patients stir it into a hot beverage like coffee, or tea, or into a hot soup. Use it to stir fry your vegetables, or to fry your eggs. Use it any place you would have used a different kind of fat.

Strategy #4: Reduce Your Stress

Stress does real damage to the brain in a variety of ways, and it would be wise to consider that even if you don't *think* you're under stress, our

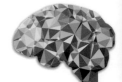

bodies recognize stress differently than we do, so there's a good chance that you are.

Here are some places to look:

- Do you work more than 40 hours per week?
- Have you taken a vacation (no work, at all!) in the last year that was a week or longer?
- Are you overscheduled?
- Do you get at last eight hours of sleep a night?
- Is the TV or radio constantly going in your house? (Noise is stressful.)
- Do you watch the news every night?
- Do you spend more than two hours a day looking at screens (TVs, computers, etc.?
- Do you travel a lot? (Sitting for long periods of time, large crowds, foreign germs, noise, restaurants, all contribute to stress.)
- Do you eat a lot of sugar, carbs, or processed foods?
- Do you exercise *too much* (more than two hours at a time more than three or four times per week)?
- And, most importantly, do you overthink or worry, creating your own stress?

The best solution for stress (other than just making sure you get enough sleep, cutting out all that travel, etc.) is meditation. And before you dismiss meditation as some New Agey practice, consider that there are huge amounts of research on its health benefits, and the research continues. A large part of that is because meditation helps with stress and our reactions to stress. It has been shown in studies directly related to cognitive function that starting a meditation or yoga practice will help your brain.[184] So if you have never experienced meditation, have an open mind and give it a try.

It's helpful to find a meditation teacher, but if that's not feasible the internet can easily support you in your practice.

Here is an easy form that I've taught my patients for years:

> Either sit or lay down comfortably in a place that is quiet and where you won't be disturbed for twenty minutes or more. Close your eyes and notice how you're breathing. Are you breathing in "spikes", which people often do when they're stressed, or are you breathing in "circles", with one breath moving smoothly into the next? Just observe for a few breaths what is occurring.

> Then, if you're not already there, bring your breathing to a "circle", with one breath moving smoothly into the next. Focus on the sound of your breath.

> You'll notice that your mind often wanders while doing this. When you realize that it has, just bring your focus back to the sound of your breath. Even if you have to do this a hundred times, it's okay. You're training your brain to do something other than thinking!

Getting a brain pattern set takes about 2–3 weeks, so practice every day if you can, and don't get frustrated (since that's just another thought as well!). You'll notice that your ability to focus will start showing up in your daily life, from improved sleep to better concentration.

Also helpful are smartphone apps — one of the best ones is called Insight Timer by Spotlight Six Software, which offers timer presets with different bells signaling the beginning, end, and intervals in the middle, it tracks your consistency, has a journal, community support, guided meditations, and lots of other great options. Another option is www.headspace.com. It's a subscription service with great meditations that lead you with

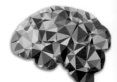

various time frames and levels. There are free ones when you first sign up, so when you need a little extra help, this can be the answer.

If you're looking for a more active form of being mindful, yoga is a great option. While it can be tempting to buy a DVD and try this at home, we'd really recommend taking some classes if you can. You will improve much more rapidly, reduce your risk of injury, and reap more benefits if you learn from a qualified instructor. After all, you wouldn't learn how to ride a bike from a DVD, would you?

Strategy #5: Sleep

Now's the time to start sleeping eight hours a night.

If you haven't been doing this already, it's probably for one of two reasons: First is a physical inability to get a full night's sleep. Adrenal fatigue — one of the side effects of poor blood sugar — is a major cause of that, so a significant number of people are able to solve their sleep problems just by taking the blood sugar solutions recommended in Strategy #1. Other common causes are sleep apnea, alcohol/tobacco use, and poor **sleep hygiene** (actions taken before bedtime that interfere with a good night's sleep). All of these are addressed in the bonus report on Sleep and Cognition, so be sure to read that if you fall into this category.

The other reason people don't sleep eight hours a night is because their lives are set up in ways that make it difficult or impossible for them to do so. You have a busy work schedule, and often find yourself working late and getting up early the next morning. You stay up late watching TV or socializing. You've got a new baby waking you up several times a night.

The only solution for people who fall into this second category is to realize just how important sleep is — just like eating or brushing your teeth or going to the toilet, this is something that must be done, or else your life will suffer — and then to arrange your life to do exactly that. Set an alarm clock to tell you when it's time to go to bed, and honor that alarm clock. If you've got kids waking you up, go to bed earlier. It sounds simple and obvious, and that's because it is. You just need to treat it as obvious and critical in order to do what needs to be done.

Strategy #6: Exercise

If you aren't already exercising, we're going to give you a variety of options to get that going. It is very clear that exercise is one of the key elements to keeping or regaining your brain health. Your brain and your body want you to *move*!

Now, contrary to popular belief, this doesn't mean you have to go to the gym every day. If you like the gym, fine, but if you don't, it really doesn't take more than a few minutes a day to reap the benefits.

That's right. One of the biggest changes in exercise science in the last decade is the understanding that short bits of intensity can cause the most improvement in the shortest amount of time. So we've picked three here have the added benefit of being particularly accessible for older people who might not have a lot of experience in this area.

Please make sure that before you start an exercise program, you check in with your doctor to make sure it's safe for you.

Exercise Option 1: 30 Minutes, Moderate-to-High Intensity

A Japanese study took middle-aged and older people for a period of more than five months and had them spend 30 minutes four times a week alternating between walking three minutes at a moderately intense pace (6–7 out of 10 on a scale of exertion) and three minutes of gentle strolling (5 sets total). They compared the results

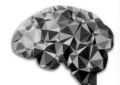

to a group that simply walked moderately (a 4 or so out of 10). At the end of the study, the group that did the intervals saw significantly improved aerobic fitness, leg strength and blood pressure readings.[185]

Not only that, but years later, when the researchers checked back in with the participants, it turns out that because of the ease of doing this and how much better they felt, over 70% of the participants had kept going, retaining and even improving their health gains!

So this exercise version is:

> **Walk at a moderate-to-high (6–7 out of 10) pace for 3 minutes, followed by gentle strolling for 3 minutes. Repeat 5 times, for a total of 30 minutes. Do this at least four times a week.**

Exercise Option 2: 12 Minutes, High Intensity

This second version was originally designed to help people with lowering their blood sugar, but it can be done by anyone. The researchers compared a group that exercised moderately for 30 minutes (walking) with a group that divided up their exercise into "snacks". The "snackers" walked as hard as they could for one minute, followed by a minute of gentle strolling, and repeated this sequence six times, for a total of 12 minutes. Some of the participants were allowed to do a minute of high-intensity upper body training using stretchy bands instead of walking. They did this mini exercise session 15–30 minutes before each meal, for a total of three times per week.

The results were amazing. The group that only walked moderately for 30 minutes didn't see any change in terms of lowering their blood sugar, but the group that did the exercise "snacks" before meal not only saw lowered blood sugar at the end of the day, but also 24 hours later!

So this exercise is:

Before each meal, walk as hard as you can for one minute, followed by gentle strolling for one minute. Repeat 6 times. You can substitute some upper-body weightlifting for a couple of the walking sessions. Repeat 4–6 times per week.

Exercise Option 3: 15 Minutes, Low-Moderate-High Intensity

A study was done on already-fit runners called "10-20-30," and the researchers noted that this form could also be perfect for inexperienced exercisers. In this study, the participants ran easy for 30 seconds (3 out of 10 intensity), accelerated moderately for 20 seconds (6 out of 10 intensity), and then ran as hard as they could for 10 seconds (9–10 out of 10). Then they rested rest at nearly a standstill for 2 minutes. They did this only 3 times a week for a total of 8 weeks.

These already-fit runners saw surprising improvements in a short time, compared to the control group who hadn't made any changes. Not only did they improve their running times significantly, but they had lowered blood pressure, lowered total cholesterol and lowered LDL cholesterol.

While it might make more sense to call this "30-20-10", here's how you do it:

Run, walk, bike or row for 30 seconds, increase to moderate pace for 20 seconds, then hard as you can for 10 seconds. Rest for 2 minutes. Repeat this 5 times. Do this 3–4 times per week.

Do you notice a theme here? It's the short, higher-intensity exercise that is helpful, so ANYTHING you do that falls within that description will help. If these examples don't appeal to you, then do something else, but just make sure you do it!

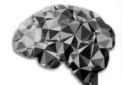

Strategy #7: Supplements

Unfortunately, given the way our society works these days, it is absolutely possible (or even likely) to have a great diet and still not get all the nutrients we need. After all, as much as we may try to eat healthy, there are so many factors working against us: our families don't want to eat those foods, restaurants no longer cater to well rounded diets like diners of years past, our produce has a shadow of the nutritional density that it had a hundred years ago. In fact, our produce has lost 85% of the minerals it used to have. Most of that occurred before 1970, so we have been on a sinking ship of health ever since.

This is where supplements come in — to help fill in those gaps. I'm going to break these down and tell you which ones are most important, under which circumstances, and why.

The B vitamins riboflavin (B2), B6, folic acid (B9), and B12 are the most important. A B complex will have all of these, but some supplements for brain health may have these optimized in relation to each other for best use. Liver is the food richest in B vitamins — a weekly staple a generation ago, but not anymore.

Amino acids like theanine, tyrosine and carnitine will help your brain function and improve your ability to burn fat for steady energy. These can be helpful when we aren't digesting protein in an ideal way.

Herbs like ginkgo and ashwaganda are helpful, but they work on a different time frame than the nutrients mentioned above. Nutrients can be felt in days. Herbs like ginkgo have a short term effect that you may feel immediately, and a long term effect that takes a few months to really kick in. These slower effects likely work by activating genes that help us resist those negative symptoms. Ashwaganda also helps our hormones, increases melatonin (sleep) and our energy. Ginseng is a good herb too, but finding quality ginkgo is hard and expensive.

Here are the rest of the good ideas: If you are or have been on a statin drug, CoQ10 is even more important for you than it already is for everyone else as we age.

Vitamin D is a vitamin that the majority of us are deficient in these days since the animals we raise often are indoors. It has a tremendous number of uses in the body as well as the brain, so I highly recommend using a vitamin A and D or D and K2 supplement.

Everyone has heard of fish oil. Unless you eat fish once or twice a week, taking a fish oil supplement is a good idea — and as one patient pointed out to me, it's cheaper than buying fish these days. Also from the sea, seaweed is your best source of iodine because it also contains every single trace mineral. However, simple iodine supplements do exist if you can't stand the idea of seaweed.

Copper and zinc can be taken as supplements or you can eat some liver each week (copper) and oysters every other week (zinc).

28-Day Plan

This 28-day Plan is designed to have you introduce one new element a week, creating a foundation on which to build your brain health. You don't have to be perfect at this, you just have to get it going. We'd recommend you start like this:

WEEK 1: Start reducing your sugar and carbohydrate intake. THIS IS VITAL. Cut down to 100 grams of carbs per day (or 60 grams per day plus vegetables), and make sure you're getting some form of fat with every meal (from coconut oil, fish,

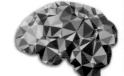

fatty plants like nuts and avocados, or naturally raised meat/ eggs/dairy; NOT from trans fats or commercially prepared vegetable oils). And finally, make sure you eat every three hours or before you're hungry. You may notice a difference in how you feel already in this first week! For a more comprehensive guide on managing blood sugar, visit http:// smartbloodsugar.com/

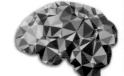

WEEK 2: Start removing fake food from your diet. Read labels. Do you recognize everything on that label? No? Then it's probably not real food. Having spent the last week cutting down your carbs, this will hopefully be much easier than you might have expected a week ago. A few other questions to ask are:

- "Would your grandmother recognize this food?"
- "Is this food a fake substitute of another food?" (like margarine for butter, or Cool Whip for real whipped cream, powdered flavoring for real herbs, etc.)
- "Is this food designed to save you time?" (frozen meals, drinkable yogurts, instant oatmeal, food designed to eat in cars, etc.)

WEEK 3: Start some exercise. You'll notice in these examples that they don't take a lot of time, and the benefits come quite quickly. Variety is also a key. Do these intervals, but perhaps add a yoga class in on other days.

WEEK 4: Start managing stress. Begin to practice the breathing exercise outlined here, and remember that it takes 2–3 weeks to get a brain pattern going. Start attending a beginner's yoga class. Start noticing where you're

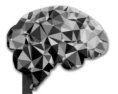

overthinking some issues, or where you're adding more drama to something than necessary. If you haven't been getting eight hours of sleep a night, arrange your life to do that starting now.

Now, you might be motivated to add in some more elements, like taking some supplements, or really starting to manage your sleep. Go for it! There are many things to take on to get your brain back on track and all of that will help!

Conclusion

Recall all the way back to the beginning of this book, in the introduction, when we talked about
Dr. Bredesen's study. Ten people with cognitive impairment were given some lifestyle changes to make, and nine of them were able to reverse their diagnosis. Among them was a 69-year old entrepreneur who had noted symptoms for 11 years, ever since he began forgetting the combination for his locker. Starting in 2003, he got tested regularly for Alzheimer's and had all the signs of it, including the APOEe4 genetic version. He struggled with recognizing faces at work, and had to have his assistants help him with his daily schedule. He lost a lifelong ability to add up columns of numbers in his head, and in one incident was several chapters into a book before he realized he had already read it previously.

In six months, he, his wife, and his co-workers all saw improvement:

> He lost 10 pounds. He was able to recognize faces at work unlike before, was able to remember his daily schedule, and was able to function at work without difficulty. He was also noted to be quicker with his responses. His ability to add columns of numbers rapidly in his head returned. His wife pointed out that, although he had clearly shown improvement, the more striking effect was that he had been accelerating in his decline over the prior year or two, and this had been completely halted.

Dr. Bredesen noted right in the study that not everyone could do everything. In fact, the two biggest complaints were the diet and lifestyle changes and the amount of pills to take. However, all the patients were acutely aware of their condition and that their prognosis was poor and their condition considered untreatable.

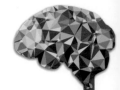

Dr. Bredesen concludes:

> Results from the 10 patients reported here suggest that memory loss in patients with subjective cognitive impairment, mild cognitive impairment, and at least the early phase of Alzheimer's disease, may be reversed, and improvement sustained, with the therapeutic program described here.

If they can do it, so can you.

References

1. Wheeler, Mark."Memory loss associated with Alzheimer's reversed for first time." *UCLA Newsroom* (October 2, 2014).

2. Bredesen, Dale E. "Reversal of cognitive decline: a novel therapeutic program." *Aging (Albany NY)* 6.9 (2014): 707.

3. Holliday, M.A.: Body composition and energy needs during growth. In: Human Growth: A Comprehensive Treatise, 2nd ea., pp. 101-117, F. Falkner, J.M. Tanner (Eds.), Plenum Press, New York, NY, 1986.

4. Ibid.

5. Murchison, Charles F., et al. "A distinct role for norepinephrine in memory retrieval." *Cell* 117.1 (2004): 131-143.

6. Bouras, Constantin, et al. "Regional distribution of neurofibrillary tangles and senile plaques in the cerebral cortex of elderly patients: a quantitative evaluation of a one-year autopsy population from a geriatric hospital." *Cerebral Cortex* 4.2 (1994): 138-150.

7. Burns A, Iliffe S. "Alzheimer's disease." *BMJ* 338 (2009): b158.

8. Plassman, Brenda L., et al. "Prevalence of dementia in the United States: the aging, demographics, and memory study." *Neuroepidemiology* 29.1-2 (2007): 125-132.

9. Payami, Haydeh, et al. "Gender difference in apolipoprotein E-associated risk for familial Alzheimer disease: a possible clue to the higher incidence of Alzheimer disease in women." *American journal of human genetics* 58.4 (1996): 803.

10. Alzheimer's Association. "2010 Alzheimer's disease facts and figures." *Alzheimer's & dementia* 6.2 (2010): 158-194.

11. "Most say they'll never get ill." United Press International. April 8, 2012.

12. "Deaths: Final Data for 2013." National vital statistics reports. Hyattsville, MD: National Center for Health Statistics. 2013. Available at http://www.cdc.gov/nchs/fastats/deaths.htm.

13. Breteler, Monique MB, et al. "Cardiovascular disease and distribution of cognitive function in elderly people: the Rotterdam Study." *BMJ* 308.6944 (1994): 1604-1608.

14. Vuorinen, Miika, et al. "Coronary Heart Disease and Cortical Thickness, Gray Matter and White Matter Lesion Volumes on MRI." (2014): e109250.

15. Muller, M., et al. "Cardiovascular disease and cognitive performance in middle-aged and elderly men." *Atherosclerosis* 190.1 (2007): 143-149.

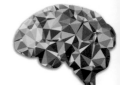

16. Knecht, Stefan, et al. "Atrial fibrillation in stroke-free patients is associated with memory impairment and hippocampal atrophy." *European heart journal* 29.17 (2008): 2125-2132.

17. Nagai, Michiaki, Satoshi Hoshide, and Kazuomi Kario. "Hypertension and dementia." *American journal of hypertension* 23.2 (2010): 116-124.

18. Peila, Rita, et al. "Reducing the risk of dementia efficacy of long-term treatment of hypertension." *Stroke* 37.5 (2006): 1165-1170.

19. Kroner, Zina. "The relationship between Alzheimer's disease and diabetes: type 3 diabetes?." *Alternative Medicine Review* 14.4 (2009): 373.

20. Suzanne, M., and Jack R. Wands. "Alzheimer's disease is type 3 diabetes — evidence reviewed." *Journal of diabetes science and technology* 2.6 (2008): 1101-1113.

21. Ohara, T., et al. "Glucose tolerance status and risk of dementia in the community The Hisayama Study." *Neurology* 77.12 (2011): 1126-1134.

22. Futamura, A., Y. Mori, and M. Kawamura. "Diabetes and dementia." *Brain Nerve* 67.6 (2015): 725-32.

23. Modrego, Pedro J., and Jaime Ferrández. "Depression in patients with mild cognitive impairment increases the risk of developing dementia of Alzheimer type: a prospective cohort study." *Archives of Neurology* 61.8 (2004): 1290-1293.

24. Bremner, J. Douglas. "Does stress damage the brain?." *Biological psychiatry* 45.7 (1999): 797-805.

25. Liu, J. Wang, X, et al. "Immobilization stress causes oxidative damage to lipid, protein, and DNA in the brain of rats." *The FASEB journal* 10.13 (1996): 1532-1538.

26. Sapolsky, Robert M. "Organismal stress and telomeric aging: An unexpected connection." *Proceedings of the National Academy of Sciences of the United States of America* 101.50 (2004): 17323-17324.

27. Cirelli, Chiara, Christina M. Gutierrez, and Giulio Tononi. "Extensive and divergent effects of sleep and wakefulness on brain gene expression." *Neuron* 41.1 (2004): 35-43.

28. Alhola, Paula, and Päivi Polo-Kantola. "Sleep deprivation: Impact on cognitive performance." *Neuropsychiatric disease and treatment* 3.5 (2007): 553.

29. Dinges, David F., et al. "Sleep deprivation and human immune function." *Advances in Neuroimmunology* 5.2 (1995): 97-110.

30. Blask, David E. "Melatonin, sleep disturbance and cancer risk." *Sleep medicine reviews* 13.4 (2009): 257-264.

31. Specker, B. L., et al. "Volumetric bone mineral density and bone size in sleep-deprived individuals." *Osteoporosis international* 18.1 (2007): 93-99.

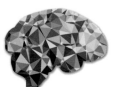

32. Lusardi, P., et al. "Effects of a restricted sleep regimen on ambulatory blood pressure monitoring in normotensive subjects." *American journal of hypertension* 9.5 (1996): 503-505.

33. Spiegel, Karine, Rachel Leproult, and Eve Van Cauter. "Impact of sleep debt on metabolic and endocrine function." *The Lancet* 354.9188 (1999): 1435-1439.

34. Taheri, Shahrad, et al. "Short sleep duration is associated with reduced leptin, elevated ghrelin, and increased body mass index." *PLoS medicine* 1.3 (2004): 210.

35. Van Dongen, Hans PA, et al. "The cumulative cost of additional wakefulness: dose-response effects on neurobehavioral functions and sleep physiology from chronic sleep restriction and total sleep deprivation." *SLEEP* 26.2 (2003): 117-129.

36. Cataldo, Janine K., Judith J. Prochaska, and Stanton A. Glantz. "Cigarette smoking is a risk factor for Alzheimer's disease: an analysis controlling for tobacco industry affiliation." *Journal of Alzheimer's disease: JAD* 19.2 (2010): 465.

37. Barnes, Deborah E., and Kristine Yaffe. "The projected effect of risk factor reduction on Alzheimer's disease prevalence." *The Lancet Neurology* 10.9 (2011): 819-828.

38. Rusanen, Minna, et al. "Heavy smoking in midlife and long-term risk of Alzheimer disease and vascular dementia." *Archives of internal medicine* 171.4 (2011): 333-339.

39. Feinkohl, I., et al. Cardiovascular risk factors and cognitive decline in older people with Type 2 diabetes. *Diabetologia* 2015 Jul; 58(7): 1637-45.

40. Laurin, Danielle, et al. "Physical activity and risk of cognitive impairment and dementia in elderly persons." *Archives of neurology* 58.3 (2001): 498-504.

41. Booth, Frank W., Christian K. Roberts, and Matthew J. Laye. "Lack of exercise is a major cause of chronic diseases." *Comprehensive Physiology* (2012).

42. Richardson, Jason R., et al. "Elevated serum pesticide levels and risk for Alzheimer disease." *JAMA neurology* 71.3 (2014): 284-290.

43. Perl, D. P., and P. F. Good. "The association of aluminum Alzheimer's disease, and neurofibrillary tangles." *Journal of neural transmission. Supplementum* 24 (1986): 205-211.

44. Walton, J. R. "Aluminum in hippocampal neurons from humans with Alzheimer's disease." *Neurotoxicology* 27.3 (2006): 385-394.

45. Tong, Ming, et al. "Nitrosamine exposure causes insulin resistance diseases: relevance to type 2 diabetes mellitus, non-alcoholic steatohepatitis, and Alzheimer's disease." *Journal of Alzheimer's disease: JAD* 17.4 (2009): 827.

46. Joutel, Anne, et al. "Cerebrovascular dysfunction and microcirculation rarefaction precede white matter lesions in a mouse genetic model of cerebral ischemic small vessel disease." *The Journal of clinical investigation* 120.2 (2010): 433.

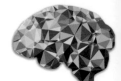

47. Mahlberg, Richard, et al. "Pineal calcification in Alzheimer's disease: an in vivo study using computed tomography." *Neurobiology of aging* 29.2 (2008): 203-209.

48. Calderon-Garciduenas, Lilian, et al. "Brain inflammation and Alzheimer's-like pathology in individuals exposed to severe air pollution." Toxicologic Pathology 32.6 (2004): 650-658.

49. "Alzheimer's Disease Genetics: Fact Sheet." NIH Publication No. 15-6424. August 2015. Available at https://www.nia.nih.gov /alzheimers/publication/alzheimers-disease-genetics-fact-sheet.

50. Gray, Shelly L., et al. "Cumulative use of strong anticholinergics and incident dementia: a prospective cohort study." *JAMA internal medicine* 175.3 (2015): 401-407.

51. Wadsworth, Emma JK, et al. "SSRIs and cognitive performance in a working sample." *Human Psychopharmacology: Clinical and Experimental* 20.8 (2005): 561-572.

52. Schaefer, Alexander, et al. "Serotonergic modulation of intrinsic functional connectivity." *Current Biology* 24.19 (2014): 2314-2318.

53. Wingo, Aliza P., et al. "Effects of lithium on cognitive performance: a meta-analysis." *The Journal of clinical psychiatry* 70.11 (2009): 1588-1597.

54. Moore, Eileen M., et al. "Increased risk of cognitive impairment in patients with diabetes is associated with metformin." *Diabetes Care* 36.10 (2013): 2981-2987.

55. Evans, Marcella A., and Beatrice A. Golomb. "Statin- Associated Adverse Cognitive Effects: Survey Results from 171 Patients." *Pharmacotherapy: The Journal of Human Pharmacology and Drug Therapy* 29.7 (2009): 800-811.

56. Gliebus, Gediminas, and Carol F. Lippa. "The Influence of β-Blockers on Delayed Memory Function in People With Cognitive Impairment." *American journal of Alzheimer's disease and other dementias* 22.1 (2007): 57-61.

57. Gazewood, John D., D. Roxanne Richards, and Karl Clebak. "Parkinson disease: an update." *Am Fam Physician* 87.4 (2013): 267-73.

58. Ciriaco, Miriam, et al. "Corticosteroid-related central nervous system side effects." *Journal of pharmacology & pharmacotherapeutics* 4.Suppl1 (2013): S94.

59. Cohen, Jay S. "Peripheral neuropathy associated with fluoroquinolones." *Annals of Pharmacotherapy* 35.12 (2001): 1540-1547.

60. De Sarro A, De Sarro G (March 2001). "Adverse reactions to fluoroquinolones. an overview on mechanistic aspects". *Curr. Med. Chem.* 8 (4): 371–84.

61. Vuurman, E. F., et al. "Seasonal allergic rhinitis and antihistamine effects on children's learning." *Annals of allergy* 71.2 (1993): 121-126.

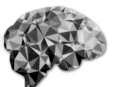

62. van Strien, Astrid M., et al. "Psychotropic medications, including short acting benzodiazepines, strongly increase the frequency of falls in elderly." *Maturitas* 74.4 (2013): 357-362.

63. de Gage, Sophie Billioti, et al. "Benzodiazepine use and risk of Alzheimer's disease: case-control study." *BMJ* 349 (2014): g5205.

64. Jayarajan, Pradeep, et al. "5-HT 6 receptor antagonist attenuates the memory deficits associated with neuropathic pain and improves the efficacy of gabapentinoids." *Pharmacological Reports* (2015).

65. Rosenberg, Russell P. "Sleep maintenance insomnia: strengths and weaknesses of current pharmacologic therapies." *Annals of Clinical Psychiatry* 18.1 (2006): 49-56.

66. Thomas, Jack. "Current drug information: Association between memory disorders and some drugs." (2012): 89.

67. Rajan, Kumar B., et al. "Cognitive impairment 18 years before clinical diagnosis of Alzheimer disease dementia." *Neurology* (2015): 10-1212.

68. Brody, JE. "Cognitive tests can help ease fears about dementia, Alzheimer's disease." *Houston Chronicle.* June 19, 2015.

69. Ohio State University: Wexner Medical Center. SAGE: A Test to Detect Signs of Alzheimer's and Dementia. Available at http://wexnermedical.osu.edu/patient-care/healthcare-services/brain-spine-neuro/memory-disorders/sage#SAGE%20Test.

70. Alzheimer's Reading Room. The Mini-Cog Test for Alzheimer's and Dementia. Available at http://www.alzheimersreadingroom.com/2009/03/mini-cog-test-for-alzheimers-and.html.

71. Alzheimer's Society. Mini-Mental State Exam. Available at http://www.alzheimers.org.uk/site/scripts/documents_info.php?documentID=121.

72. MoCA. Montreal Cognitive Assessment. Available at http://www.mocatest.org/.

73. 2015 Alzheimer's Disease Facts and Figures. Alzheimer's Association. http://www.alz.org/facts/.

74. Potter, Guy G., Douglas R. McQuoid, and David C. Steffens. "Appetite loss and neurocognitive deficits in late -life depression." International journal of geriatric psychiatry 30.6 (2015): 647-654.

75. Rémond, Didier, et al. "Understanding the gastrointestinal tract of the elderly to develop dietary solutions that prevent malnutrition." *Oncotarget* 6.16 (2015): 13858.

76. Squire LR. *Fundamental neuroscience.* 2nd. ed. San Diego, CA. (2003): xix, 1426.

77.   Kanoski, Scott E., and Terry L. Davidson. "Western diet consumption and cognitive impairment: links to hippocampal dysfunction and obesity." *Physiology & behavior* 103.1 (2011): 59-68.

78.   Agrawal, Rahul, and Fernando Gomez- Pinilla. "'Metabolic syndrome'in the brain: deficiency in omega- 3 fatty acid exacerbates dysfunctions in insulin receptor signalling and cognition." *The Journal of physiology* 590.10 (2012): 2485-2499.

79.   De La Monte, S. M. "Metabolic derangements mediate cognitive impairment and Alzheimer's disease: role of peripheral insulin-resistance diseases." *Panminerva medica* 54.3 (2012): 171-178.

80.   Guzmán, Manuel, and Cristina Blázquez. "Ketone body synthesis in the brain: possible neuroprotective effects." *Prostaglandins, Leukotrienes and Essential Fatty Acids* 70.3 (2004): 287-292.

81.   The Ketogenic Diet Center, Johns Hopkins Medicine. Available at http://www.hopkinsmedicine.org/neurology_neurosurgery/centers_clinics/epilepsy/ pediatric_epilepsy/ketogenic_diet.html.

82.   Papamandjaris, Andrea A., Diane E. MacDougall, and Peter JH Jones. "Medium chain fatty acid metabolism and energy expenditure: obesity treatment implications." *Life sciences* 62.14 (1998): 1203-1215.

83.   Guzmán, Manuel, and Cristina Blázquez. "Ketone body synthesis in the brain: possible neuroprotective effects." *Prostaglandins, leukotrienes and essential fatty acids* 70.3 (2004): 287-292.

84.   Trivedi, Madhukar H., et al. "Exercise as an augmentation treatment for nonremitted major depressive disorder: a randomized, parallel dose comparison." *Journal of Clinical Psychiatry* 72.5 (2011): 677.

85.   Babyak, Michael, et al. "Exercise treatment for major depression: maintenance of therapeutic benefit at 10 months." *Psychosomatic Medicine* 62.5 (2000): 633-638.

86.   Quistorff, Bjørn, Niels H. Secher, and Johannes J. Van Lieshout. "Lactate fuels the human brain during exercise." *The FASEB Journal* 22.10 (2008): 3443-3449.

87.   Wyss, Matthias T., et al. "In vivo evidence for lactate as a neuronal energy source." *The Journal of Neuroscience* 31.20 (2011): 7477-7485.

88.   Lautenschlager, Nicola T., et al. "Effect of physical activity on cognitive function in older adults at risk for Alzheimer disease: a randomized trial." *Jama* 300.9 (2008): 1027-1037.

89.   Abbott RD, White LR, Ross GW, Masaki KH, Curb JD, Petrovitch H. Walking and dementia in physically capable elderly men. *JAMA*. 292.12 (2004):1447-1453

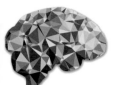

90. Alosco, Michael L., et al. "Decreases in daily physical activity predict acute decline in attention and executive function in heart failure." *Journal of Cardiac Failure* 21.4 (2015): 339-346.

91. Wilcox, Sara, et al. "Perceptions and beliefs about the role of physical activity and nutrition on brain health in older adults." *The Gerontologist* 49.S1 (2009): S61-S71.

92. Cotman, Carl W., Nicole C. Berchtold, and Lori-Ann Christie. "Exercise builds brain health: key roles of growth factor cascades and inflammation." *Trends in Neurosciences* 30.9 (2007): 464-472.

93. Smith, J. Carson, et al. "Physical activity and brain function in older adults at increased risk for Alzheimer's disease." *Brain sciences* 3.1 (2013): 54-83.

94. Forbes, Scott C., et al. "Exercise interventions for maintaining cognitive function in cognitively healthy people in late life." *The Cochrane Library* (2015).

95. Liu-Ambrose, Teresa, et al. "Resistance training and executive functions: a 12-month randomized controlled trial." *Archives of internal medicine* 170.2 (2010): 170-178.

96. Diamond, Adele. "Effects of Physical Exercise on Executive Functions: Going beyond Simply Moving to Moving with Thought." *Annals of sports medicine and research* 2.1 (2015): 1011.

97. Agudelo, Leandro Z., et al. "Skeletal muscle PGC-1α1 modulates kynurenine metabolism and mediates resilience to stress-induced depression." *Cell* 159.1 (2014): 33-45.

98. Grosse, Susan J. "Brain Gym in the Pool." *International Journal of Aquatic Research & Education* 7.1 (2013).

99. Bento, Paulo Cesar Barauce, et al. "The Effects of a Water-based Training on Static and Dynamic Balance of Older Women." *Rejuvenation research ja* (2015).

100. Nouchi, Rui, et al. "Brain training game improves executive functions and processing speed in the elderly: a randomized controlled trial." (2012): e29676.

101. Matthews, Steve. "Dementia and the Power of Music Therapy." *Bioethics* (2015).

102. Marioni, Riccardo E., et al. "Active cognitive lifestyle associates with cognitive recovery and a reduced risk of cognitive decline." *Journal of Alzheimer's Disease* 28.1 (2012): 223.

103. Ferreira, Nicola, et al. "Associations between cognitively stimulating leisure activities, cognitive function and age- related cognitive decline." *International journal of geriatric psychiatry* 30.4 (2015): 422-430.

104. Finn, Maurice, and Skye McDonald. "Computerised cognitive training for older persons with mild cognitive impairment: a pilot study using a randomised controlled trial design." *Brain Impairment* 12.03 (2011): 187-199.

105. Kueider, Alexandra M., et al. "Computerized cognitive training with older adults: a systematic review." *PloS one* 7.7 (2012): e40588..

106. Cacioppo, John T., and Louise C. Hawkley. "Perceived social isolation and cognition." *Trends in Cognitive Sciences* 13.10 (2009): 447-454.

107. Holt-Lunstad, Julianne, et al. "Loneliness and Social Isolation as Risk Factors for Mortality A Meta-Analytic Review." *Perspectives on Psychological Science* 10.2 (2015): 227-237.

108. Op. Cit. Cacioppo.

109. Fratiglioni, Laura, et al. "Influence of social network on occurrence of dementia: a community-based longitudinal study." *The Lancet* 355.9212 (2000): 1315-1319.

110. Xie, Lulu, et al. "Sleep drives metabolite clearance from the adult brain." *Science* 342.6156 (2013): 373-377.

111. Brown, Ritchie E., et al. "Control of sleep and wakefulness." *Physiological Reviews* 92.3 (2012): 1087-1187.

112. Zaregarizi, Mohammad, et al. "Acute changes in cardiovascular function during the onset period of daytime sleep: comparison to lying awake and standing." *Journal of Applied Physiology* 103.4 (2007): 1332-1338.

113. Naska, Androniki, et al. "Siesta in healthy adults and coronary mortality in the general population." *Archives of Internal Medicine* 167.3 (2007): 296-301.

114. Walker, M. P., et al. "Sleep-dependent motor memory plasticity in the human brain." *Neuroscience* 133.4 (2005): 911-917.

115. Vertes, Robert P. "Memory consolidation in sleep: dream or reality." *Neuron* 44.1 (2004): 135-148.

116. Robinson, Jo. "Breeding the Nutrition Out of Our Food." *The New York Times,* May 25 (2013).

117. Ahmed, Tanvir, and Nadim Haboubi. "Assessment and Management of Nutrition in Older People and Its Importance to Health." *Clinical Interventions in Aging* 5 (2010): 207–216.

118. Rickman, Joy C., Diane M. Barrett, and Christine M. Bruhn. "Nutritional comparison of fresh, frozen and canned fruits and vegetables. Part 1. Vitamins C and B and phenolic compounds." *Journal of the Science of Food and Agriculture* 87.6 (2007): 930-944.

119. Dahm, Daniel. "Casselberry mom refused to take child to hospital over vegan beliefs." *ClickOrlando.com,* August 6 (2014). Web.

120. Kocaoglu, Celebi, et al. "Cerebral atrophy in a vitamin B12-deficient infant of a vegetarian mother." *Journal of Health, Population, and Nutrition* 32.2 (2014): 367.

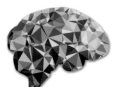

121. LeBlanc, Erin S., and Roger Chou. "Vitamin D and Falls — Fitting New Data With Current Guidelines." *JAMA Internal Medicine* 175.5 (2015): 712-713.

122. Morris, Martha Savaria. "The role of B vitamins in preventing and treating cognitive impairment and decline." *Advances in Nutrition: An International Review Journal* 3.6 (2012): 801-812.

123. Qin, Bo, et al. "B vitamin intake in early adulthood and cognition in late midlife: CARDIA." *The FASEB Journal* 27.1_MeetingAbstracts (2013): 840-2.

124. Sinigaglia-Coimbra, Rita, Antonio Carlos Lopes, and Cicero G. Coimbra. "Riboflavin Deficiency, Brain Function, and Health." *Handbook of Behavior, Food and Nutrition*. Springer New York, 2011. 2427-2449.

125. Morris, Martha Savaria. "The role of B vitamins in preventing and treating cognitive impairment and decline." *Advances in Nutrition: An International Review Journal* 3.6 (2012): 801-812.

126. Snyder, Heather M., et al. "Vascular contributions to cognitive impairment and dementia including Alzheimer's disease." *Alzheimer's & Dementia* (2014).

127. Smith, A. David, et al. "Homocysteine-lowering by B vitamins slows the rate of accelerated brain atrophy in mild cognitive impairment: a randomized controlled trial." *PLoS ONE* 5.9 (2010): e12244.

128. Bryan, Janet, Eva Calvaresi, and Donna Hughes. "Short-term folate, vitamin B-12 or vitamin B-6 supplementation slightly affects memory performance but not mood in women of various ages." *The Journal of Nutrition* 132.6 (2002): 1345-1356.

129. Mitchell, E. Siobhan, Nelly Conus, and Jim Kaput. "B vitamin polymorphisms and behavior: Evidence of associations with neurodevelopment, depression, schizophrenia, bipolar disorder and cognitive decline." *Neuroscience & Biobehavioral Reviews* 47 (2014): 307-320.

130. Yajnik, Chittaranjan S., et al. "Oral vitamin B12 supplementation reduces plasma total homocysteine concentration in women in India." *Asia Pacific Journal of Clinical Nutrition* 16.1 (2007): 103-9.

131. Malouf, Reem, and John Grimley Evans. "Folic acid with or without vitamin B12 for the prevention and treatment of healthy elderly and demented people." *The Cochrane Library* (2008).

132. Douaud, Gwenaëlle, et al. "Preventing Alzheimer's disease-related gray matter atrophy by B-vitamin treatment." *Proceedings of the National Academy of Sciences* 110.23 (2013): 9523-9528.

133. Erickson, Kirk I., et al. "Greater intake of vitamins B6 and B12 spares gray matter in healthy elderly: A voxel-based morphometry study." *Brain Research* 1199 (2008): 20-26.

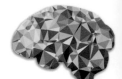

134. Smith, A. David, et al. "Homocysteine-lowering by B vitamins slows the rate of accelerated brain atrophy in mild cognitive impairment: a randomized controlled trial." *PLoS ONE* 5.9 (2010): e12244.

135. "Health Conditions" *VitaminDCouncil.org.* Vitamin D Council. Available at http://www.vitamindcouncil.org/health-conditions/cognitive-impairment/.

136. Wilkins, Consuelo H., et al. "Vitamin D deficiency is associated with worse cognitive performance and lower bone density in older African Americans." *Journal of the National Medical Association* 101.4 (2009): 349.

137. Wilkins, Consuelo H., et al. "Vitamin D deficiency is associated with low mood and worse cognitive performance in older adults." *The American Journal of Geriatric Psychiatry* 14.12 (2006): 1032-1040.

138. Jorde, Rolf, et al. "Neuropsychological function in relation to serum parathyroid hormone and serum 25–hydroxyvitamin D levels." *Journal of Neurology* 253.4 (2006): 464-470.

139. Lee, David M., et al. "Association between 25-hydroxyvitamin D levels and cognitive performance in middle-aged and older European men." *Journal of Neurology, Neurosurgery & Psychiatry* 80.7 (2009): 722-729.

140. Llewellyn, David J., et al. "Vitamin D and risk of cognitive decline in elderly persons." *Archives of Internal Medicine* 170.13 (2010): 1135-1141.

141. Llewellyn, David J., Kenneth M. Langa, and Iain A. Lang. "Serum 25-hydroxyvitamin D concentration and cognitive impairment." *Journal of Geriatric Psychiatry and Neurology* 22.3 (2009): 188-195.

142. Miller, Joshua W. "Vitamin D and cognitive function in older adults Are we concerned about vitamin D-mentia?." *Neurology* 74.1 (2010): 13-15.

143. Przybelski, Robert J., and Neil C. Binkley. "Is vitamin D important for preserving cognition? A positive correlation of serum 25-hydroxyvitamin D concentration with cognitive function." *Archives of Biochemistry and Biophysics* 460.2 (2007): 202-205.

144. Seamans, K. M., et al. "Vitamin D status and measures of cognitive function in healthy older European adults." *European Journal of Clinical Nutrition* 64.10 (2010): 1172-1178.

145. Van der Schaft, J., et al. "The association between vitamin D and cognition: a systematic review." *Ageing Research Reviews* 12.4 (2013): 1013-1023.

146. Anglin, Rebecca ES, et al. "Vitamin D deficiency and depression in adults: systematic review and meta-analysis." *The British Journal of Psychiatry* 202.2 (2013): 100-107.

147. Hallahan, Brian, et al. "Omega-3 fatty acid supplementation in patients with recurrent self-harm." *The British Journal of Psychiatry* 190.2 (2007): 118-122.

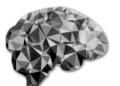

148. Frangou, Sophia, Michael Lewis, and Paul McCrone. "Efficacy of ethyl-eicosapentaenoic acid in bipolar depression: randomised double-blind placebo-controlled study." *The British Journal of Psychiatry* 188.1 (2006): 46-50.

149. Raeder, Maria Baroy, et al. "Associations between cod liver oil use and symptoms of depression: the Hordaland Health Study." *Journal of Affective Disorders* 101.1 (2007): 245-249.

150. Pajonk, Frank-Gerald, et al. "Cognitive decline correlates with low plasma concentrations of copper in patients with mild to moderate Alzheimer's disease." *Journal of Alzheimer's disease: JAD* 8.1 (2005): 23-27.

151. Klevay, Leslie M. "Alzheimer's disease as copper deficiency." *Medical Hypotheses* 70.4 (2008): 802-807.

152. Pan, Enhui, et al. "Vesicular zinc promotes presynaptic and inhibits postsynaptic long-term potentiation of mossy fiber-CA3 synapse." *Neuron* 71.6 (2011): 1116-1126.

153. Warthon-Medina, M., et al. "The relationship between zinc intake and indices of cognitive function: A systematic review and meta-analyses." *Proceedings of the Nutrition Society* 72.OCE4 (2013): E210.

154. Fosmire, Gary J. "Zinc toxicity." *The American journal of clinical nutrition* 51.2 (1990): 225-227.

155. Brewer, George J. "Copper excess, zinc deficiency, and cognition loss in Alzheimer's disease." *Biofactors* 38.2 (2012): 107-113.

156. Nobre, Anna C., Anling Rao, and Gail N. Owen. "L-theanine, a natural constituent in tea, and its effect on mental state." *Asia Pacific Journal Clinical Nutrition* 17.suppl 1 (2008): 167-168.

157. Gomez-Ramirez, Manuel, et al. "The effects of L-theanine on alpha-band oscillatory brain activity during a visuo-spatial attention task." *Brain Topography* 22.1 (2009): 44-51.

158. Mahoney, Caroline R., et al. "Tyrosine supplementation mitigates working memory decrements during cold exposure." *Physiology & Behavior* 92.4 (2007): 575-582.

159. Colzato, Lorenza S., et al. "Working memory reloaded: tyrosine repletes updating in the N-back task." *Frontiers in Behavioral Neuroscience* 7 (2013).

160. Onofrj, Marco, et al. "Acetyl-L-carnitine: from a biological curiosity to a drug for the peripheral nervous system and beyond." *Expert Review of Neurotherapeutics* 13.8 (2013): 925-936.

161. Malaguarnera, Michele, et al. "Acetyl L-carnitine (ALC) treatment in elderly patients with fatigue." *Archives of Gerontology and Geriatrics* 46.2 (2008): 181-190.

162. Zhou, Peng, et al. "Acetyl-L-carnitine attenuates homocysteine-induced Alzheimer-like histopathological and behavioral abnormalities." *Rejuvenation Research* 14.6 (2011): 669-679.

163. Zana, Marianna, Zoltán Janka, and János Kálmán. "Oxidative stress: a bridge between Down's syndrome and Alzheimer's disease." *Neurobiology of Aging* 28.5 (2007): 648-676.

164. Ribas, Graziela S., Carmen R. Vargas, and Moacir Wajner. "L-carnitine supplementation as a potential antioxidant therapy for inherited neurometabolic disorders." *Gene* 533.2 (2014): 469-476.

165. Dhanasekaran, Muralikrishnan, and Jun Ren. "The emerging role of coenzyme Q-10 in aging, neurodegeneration, cardiovascular disease, cancer and diabetes mellitus." *Current Neurovascular Research* 2.5 (2005): 447-459.

166. Langsjoen, Peter H., and Alena M. Langsjoen. "The clinical use of HMG CoA -reductase inhibitors and the associated depletion of coenzyme Q10. A review of animal and human publications." *Biofactors* 18.1-4 (2003): 101-111.

167. Ayer, Anita, Peter Macdonald, and Roland Stocker. "CoQ10 Function and Role in Heart Failure and Ischemic Heart Disease." *Annual Review of Nutrition* 35.0 (2015): 175-213

168. Nazar, Abdullah. "Beauty is now more than skin deep — the emergence of cosmeceuticals." *Public Health* 16 (2014): 46.

169. Kale, Mayura A., Suparna M. Bindu, and Pratima Khadkikar. "Role of Antioxidants and Nutrition in Oxidative Stress: A Review." *International Journal of Applied Pharmaceutics,* 7.1 (2015)

170. Ajith, T. A., and G. Padmajanair. "Mitochondrial pharmaceutics: A new therapeutic strategy to ameliorate oxidative stress in Alzheimer's disease." *Current Aging Science* 8.3 (2015).

171. Galasko, Douglas R., et al. "Antioxidants for Alzheimer disease: a randomized clinical trial with cerebrospinal fluid biomarker measures." *Archives of Neurology* 69.7 (2012): 836-841.

172. Kaschel, R. "Specific memory effects of Ginkgo biloba extract EGb 761 in middle-aged healthy volunteers." *Phytomedicine* 18.14 (2011): 1202-1207.

173. Solfrizzi, Vincenzo, and Francesco Panza. "Plant-Based Nutraceutical Interventions against Cognitive Impairment and Dementia: Meta-Analytic Evidence of Efficacy of a Standardized Gingko biloba Extract." *Journal of Alzheimer's Disease: JAD* 43.2 (2015): 605-611.

174. Chandrasekhar, K., Jyoti Kapoor, and Sridhar Anishetty. "A prospective, randomized double-blind, placebo-controlled study of safety and efficacy of a high-concentration full-spectrum extract of ashwagandha root in reducing stress and anxiety in adults." *Indian Journal of Psychological Medicine* 34.3 (2012): 255.

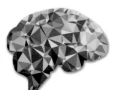

175. Chandrasekhar, K., Jyoti Kapoor, and Sridhar Anishetty. "A prospective, randomized double-blind, placebo-controlled study of safety and efficacy of a high-concentration full-spectrum extract of ashwagandha root in reducing stress and anxiety in adults." *Indian journal of psychological medicine* 34.3 (2012): 255.

176. Calabrese, Carlo, et al. "Effects of a standardized Bacopa monnieri extract on cognitive performance, anxiety, and depression in the elderly: a randomized, double-blind, placebo-controlled trial." *The Journal of Alternative and Complementary Medicine* 14.6 (2008): 707-713.

177. Stough, Con, et al. "Examining the nootropic effects of a special extract of Bacopa monniera on human cognitive functioning: 90 day double-blind placebo-controlled randomized trial." *Phytotherapy Research* 22.12 (2008): 1629-1634.

178. Uabundit, Nongnut, et al. "Cognitive enhancement and neuroprotective effects of Bacopa monnieri in Alzheimer's disease model." *Journal of ethnopharmacology* 127.1 (2010): 26-31.

179. Henderson, Samuel T. "Ketone bodies as a therapeutic for Alzheimer's disease." *Neurotherapeutics* 5.3 (2008): 470-480.

180. Reger, Mark A., et al. "Effects of β-hydroxybutyrate on cognition in memory-impaired adults." *Neurobiology of Aging* 25.3 (2004): 311-314.

181. Henderson, S. T. "High carbohydrate diets and Alzheimer's disease." *Medical hypotheses* 62.5 (2004): 689

182. Ibid.

183. Reger, M. A., et al. "Effects of beta-hydroxybutyrate on cognition in memory-impaired adults." *Neurobiol Aging* 25.3 (2004): 311-4.

184. Gard, Tim, Britta K. Hölzel, and Sara W. Lazar. "The potential effects of meditation on age-related cognitive decline: a systematic review." *Annals of the New York Academy of Sciences* 1307.1 (2014): 89-103.

185. Nemoto, Ken-ichi, et al. "Effects of high-intensity interval walking training on physical fitness and blood pressure in middle-aged and older people." *Mayo Clinic Proceedings*. Vol. 82. No. 7. Elsevier, 2007.

186. Francois, Monique E., et al. "'Exercise snacks' before meals: a novel strategy to improve glycaemic control in individuals with insulin resistance." *Diabetologia* 57.7 (2014): 1437-1445.